— THE EASY —
Air Fryer Cookbook

HEALTHY, EVERYDAY RECIPES FOR PEOPLE WITH DIABETES

WYSS & MOORE

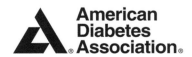

American Diabetes Association

Associate Publisher, Books, Abe Ogden; *Director, Book Operations,* Victor Van Beuren; *Managing Editor, Books,* John Clark; *Associate Director, Book Marketing,* Annette Reape; *Acquisitions Editor,* Jaclyn Konich; *Senior Manager, Book Editing,* Lauren Wilson; *Editor,* Abigail Yeager; *Composition,* Circle Graphics; *Cover Design,* Vis-a-Vis; *Printer,* Versa Press.

Printed in the United States of America
3 5 7 9 10 8 6 4 2

The suggestions and information contained in this publication are generally consistent with the *Standards of Medical Care in Diabetes* and other policies of the American Diabetes Association, but they do not represent the policy or position of the Association or any of its boards or committees. Reasonable steps have been taken to ensure the accuracy of the information presented. However, the American Diabetes Association cannot ensure the safety or efficacy of any product or service described in this publication. Individuals are advised to consult a physician or other appropriate healthcare professional before undertaking any diet or exercise program or taking any medication referred to in this publication. Professionals must use and apply their own professional judgment, experience, and training and should not rely solely on the information contained in this publication before prescribing any diet, exercise, or medication. The American Diabetes Association—its officers, directors, employees, volunteers, and members—assumes no responsibility or liability for personal or other injury, loss, or damage that may result from the suggestions or information in this publication.

Madelyn Wheeler conducted the internal review of this book to ensure that it meets American Diabetes Association guidelines.

⊗ The paper in this publication meets the requirements of the ANSI Standard Z39. 48-1992 (permanence of paper).

ADA titles may be purchased for business or promotional use or for special sales. To purchase more than 50 copies of this book at a discount, or for custom editions of this book with your logo, contact the American Diabetes Association at the address below or at booksales@diabetes.org.

American Diabetes Association
2451 Crystal Drive, Suite 900
Arlington, VA 22202

DOI: 10.2337/9781580407038

Library of Congress Cataloging-in-Publication Data

Names: Wyss, Roxanne, author. | Moore, Kathy, 1954- author. | American Diabetes Association, publisher.
Title: The easy air fryer cookbook : healthy, everyday recipes for people with diabetes / Roxanne Wyss and Kathy Moore.
Description: Arlington : American Diabetes Association, [2019] | Includes index.
Identifiers: LCCN 2019004493 | ISBN 9781580407038 (softcover : alk. paper)
Subjects: LCSH: Diabetes--Diet therapy--Recipes. | Hot air frying. | LCGFT: Cookbooks.
Classification: LCC RC662 .W97 2019 | DDC 641.5/6314--dc23
LC record available at https://lccn.loc.gov/2019004493

Contents

81 Vegetables and Sides

Dedication

We dedicate this book to all the families who gather at the dinner table for memorable, nutritious meals and in celebration of our 30-plus years of working with small appliances and creating delicious recipes for families to enjoy.

Diabetes Nutrition 101

If you've just been diagnosed with diabetes or prediabetes, you're probably wondering what, when, and how much you need to eat. You may be surprised to hear that when it comes to diabetes nutrition, there is no "one-size-fits-all" approach—no "diabetes diet" or perfect amount of nutrients (protein, fat, or even carbohydrates) that is right for every person with diabetes. Diabetes affects people of all ages, across all cultures, with all different health backgrounds, eating preferences, and budgets. So it makes sense that there is a variety of eating patterns that can help people manage diabetes. The eating pattern you follow should be personalized to meet your needs, fit your lifestyle, and help you achieve your health goals. With the help of your healthcare team, you can create an eating plan that will work best for you. A Registered Dietitian Nutritionist (RDN) or Certified Diabetes Educator (CDE) in particular can help you manage your diabetes or prediabetes through diet and lifestyle changes. Ask your primary care provider for a referral if an RDN or CDE is not already a part of your care team. In most cases, appointments with an RDN or CDE are covered by insurance.

What Is an Eating Pattern?

"Eating pattern" is simply a term used to describe the foods or groups of foods that a person chooses to eat on a daily basis over time. Examples of eating patterns are vegetarian/vegan, low-carb, low-fat, or Mediterranean-style.

When choosing an eating pattern with your diabetes care team, look for a plan that you feel you can incorporate into your lifestyle and follow long term. It is important for your eating plan to fit your needs, so you can stick to one pattern or implement strategies from a variety of patterns. Remember to take your food likes and dislikes, time constraints, food access, and budget into account as well.

But no matter which eating pattern you choose, there are a few tips you can focus on to make managing your diabetes easier:

- **Eat nonstarchy vegetables**
  - Nonstarchy vegetables are low in calories and carbohydrates and high in essential vitamins and minerals. These include greens (lettuce, spinach, kale, arugula), asparagus, beets, Brussels sprouts, broccoli, cauliflower, carrots, celery, cucumber, mushrooms, onions, peppers, tomatoes, and zucchini.

- **Limit added sugars and refined grains**
  - Added sugars are the sweeteners (such as sugar, corn syrup, brown sugar, honey, maple syrup, and others) added to some foods when they are processed. Added sugars are found in many foods, but a few major sources of added sugars are sodas and energy drinks, fruit drinks,

baked goods, and candy and desserts (such as ice cream). Refined grains include white or highly processed flours and the products made with them (such as white breads and pastas and many baked goods).

- **Choose whole foods over highly processed foods as often as possible**
  - Whole foods are foods that are as close to their natural form as possible and have had very little processing. Whole foods—such as fresh or frozen fruits and vegetables, beans, whole grains, and fresh meats, poultry, and seafood—provide nutrients that are often removed from processed foods.

- **Choose zero-calorie drinks**
  - If you're thirsty, the best choice is always water. Unsweetened coffee or tea, sparkling water, or flavored waters (made without sugar) are also good choices if you are looking for something more interesting. Try to avoid sugary drinks such as sodas, fruit-flavored drinks, energy drinks, and sweetened coffees and teas.

Common Eating Patterns to Help Manage Diabetes

Mediterranean-Style—This eating pattern emphasizes plant-based foods (vegetables, beans, nuts and seeds, fruits, and whole intact grains), fish and other seafood, and olive oil (which is the main source of fat in this eating pattern). Dairy products, eggs, and wine are included in moderation. Red meat is eaten rarely, as are sweets, added sugars, and honey. A Mediterranean-style eating pattern may reduce the risk of developing diabetes, and can help lower A1C in people with diabetes. It may also help protect against heart disease and stroke.

Vegetarian or Vegan—Both of these options are plant-based eating patterns. They are rich in vitamins, minerals, and fiber, and low in fat and cholesterol. People who follow a vegetarian eating pattern do not eat meat, poultry, fish, or seafood, though some may choose to eat eggs and/or dairy products. With a vegan eating pattern, all animal products are avoided, including dairy products, eggs, and even honey. Following a vegetarian or vegan eating pattern may help reduce the risk of diabetes, lower A1C, and promote weight loss.

Low-Fat or Very Low-Fat—These eating patterns emphasize vegetables, fruits, starches (e.g., breads/crackers, pasta, whole grains, and starchy vegetables), lean protein sources, and low-fat dairy products. A low-fat eating pattern is defined as eating less than 30% of your total calories as fat and less than 10% as saturated fat. A very low-fat eating pattern means that a person eats 70–77% carbohydrate (including a lot of fiber), 10% fat, and 13–20% protein per day. A low-fat eating pattern may promote weight loss and reduce the risk of diabetes. A very low-fat eating pattern may also help lower blood pressure.

Low-Carb or Very Low-Carb—Low-carb eating patterns emphasize vegetables that are low in carbohydrate (also known as nonstarchy vegetables)—such as salad greens, broccoli, cauliflower, cucumber, cabbage, and others. These eating patterns include fat from animal foods, oils, butter, and avocado, and protein in the form of meat, poultry, fish, shellfish, eggs, cheese, nuts, and seeds. People following a low-carb eating pattern avoid starchy and sugary foods such as pasta, rice, potatoes, bread, and sweets. Although there is no clear definition of "low-carb," people following this eating pattern generally reduce their carbohydrate intake to 26–45% of their daily calories (low-carb) or less than 26% of their daily calories (very low-carb). Low-carb eating patterns have the potential to reduce A1C, promote weight loss, and lower blood pressure.

Dietary Approaches to Stop Hypertension (DASH)—This heart-friendly eating pattern emphasizes vegetables, fruits, low-fat dairy products, whole grains, poultry, fish, and nuts. It limits saturated fat, red meat, and sugar-containing foods and beverages. It may also limit sodium. The DASH eating pattern may have the benefit of lowering blood pressure, reducing the risk of diabetes, and promoting weight loss.

With this wide selection of eating patterns available to help manage (or prevent) diabetes, you're sure to find an option that works for you!

What Are Carbs and Why Are They Important?

Carbohydrate is a readily used source of energy and the primary dietary influence on blood glucose. A food or drink that contains carbohydrate will have a greater effect on blood glucose than foods that contain protein or fat. Carbohydrate foods can be rich in dietary fiber, vitamins, and minerals and low in added sugars, fats, and sodium, but it is important to focus on the quality of carbohydrate you consume. Fruits, vegetables, beans, and whole grains contain carbohydrates, as do white breads, pastas, and soda. Carbs that come from whole, high-fiber foods are healthier choices than highly processed or sugary foods and drinks. There is not a set amount of carbs that is right for everyone with diabetes to eat each day or at each meal. Reducing total carbs or choosing higher-quality carbs can help with managing blood glucose, but people with diabetes do not need to eliminate or severely restrict carbs to stay healthy. Your carbohydrate intake is a personal decision, which will ideally be based on the personal eating plan that you create with your dietitian or healthcare team. Your healthcare team can help you set carbohydrate goals that are right for you and help you successfully manage diabetes.

Weight Loss

Weight loss can be helpful for improving blood glucose levels in people with both type 1 and type 2 diabetes and prediabetes. Losing as little as 5% of your body weight can improve diabetes management and reduce your risk for diabetes-related health problems. Strategies for weight loss include changes to your eating behaviors (especially eating fewer calories), regular exercise, or medication and weight-loss surgery. If losing weight is one of your health goals, your healthcare team can help create a weight-loss plan that is safe and appropriate for you.

Looking for a Place to Start?

A good tool to get you started on your journey with diabetes nutrition is the Diabetes Plate Method. If you haven't had a chance to discuss a meal plan with your diabetes care team yet, this meal planning method is an easy way to eat nutritious foods in reasonable portion sizes—and there's no carbohydrate counting or special equipment required! Just start with a 9-inch dinner plate, and fill half of that plate with nonstarchy vegetables (such as salad greens, carrots, broccoli, cauliflower, green beans). Then fill one-quarter of the plate with a protein food (such as chicken, turkey, fish, tofu, etc.), and you can fill the remaining one-quarter with a carb food (such as starchy vegetables like potatoes, grains, fruit, milk, or yogurt). With the Diabetes Plate Method, you can still enjoy your favorite foods (being mindful of portions, of course!) while managing your diabetes.

Quick Cooking for Healthy Living

Healthy food choices that taste great and are ready to enjoy in just minutes are a dream come true. Thanks to the new air fryers, it is possible to cook many delicious and healthy foods! This simple appliance offers numerous benefits.

What Is Air Frying?

Swirling hot air cooks the food quickly in your new air fryer. The food is placed in a wire mesh basket or on a rack and is surrounded by circulating, hot air. The hot air is moving so quickly and evenly that it insures quick cooking and a crisp, brown crust.

Benefits of Air Frying

There are several great reasons to make an air fryer your go-to kitchen appliance:

1. **Easy to use:** Just place the food in the air fryer basket, set the temperature, and the air fryer does the rest. Give the air fryer basket a shake or two midway through the cooking time and enjoy delicious, golden-brown foods.

2. **Quick:** The air fryer cooks the food in just minutes. No big oven to preheat and no deep fat to heat.

3. **Uses little or no oil:** Just a light mist of oil is all you need to add the flavor you seek. Some foods don't even need that. You can enjoy crisp and crunchy foods without the fat.

4. **Creates a brown and crispy texture:** Foods brown beautifully and get crispy in the air fryer.

5. **Cleans up easily:** Give the air fryer basket and the bottom tray a quick rinse in hot, soapy water. There's no used oil to discard like you have with traditional fryers. Most air fryers are nonstick coated and never need abrasive cleansers.

6. **Cooks a wide variety of foods:** Use the air fryer every day for a wide variety of foods—fish, poultry, meats, vegetables, eggs, fruit, and more. Breakfast, lunch, dinner, and even dessert will be done in just minutes.

Using Your Air Fryer to Create Diabetes-Friendly Dishes

Thanks to the air fryer, people with diabetes can enjoy crispy, crunchy delicacies without the added fat from deep frying. That same air fryer means everyone who enjoys a healthier diet can get a delicious meal on the table quickly and easily. Families can enjoy tasty, appealing meals even on the busiest of days when they use their air fryer. Let's get started!

Always refer to the manufacturer's directions for your particular model. The manufacturer's instructions will contain important information about the quantity of food your air fryer can hold, the temperature settings, and unique directions that should be followed.

Once you've used your air fryer a few times, you will know if the cooking times listed in the recipes in this book will work well for your particular air fryer model or if you need to adjust the times so the food is cooked a little less or a little more, to suit your preference. You may also find that you prefer to adjust the temperature setting slightly up or down for your particular unit. The recipes that follow were carefully tested in a variety of air fryers, but they are mainly guidelines. Each unit may operate slightly differently.

Be careful. The air fryer will be hot during use.

How to Use Your Air Fryer:

1. Place the food in the air fryer basket. Do not crowd the food. It is always better to cook two small batches than one larger basketful. The actual volume that will work well in a basket varies by air fryer model.

2. Set the temperature and the time. The temperature will often be set between 350°F and 400°F. Most air fryers have a built-in timer and operate only when the timer is set.

3. Shake the basket to rearrange the food midway through the cooking time. Some foods may require frequent shaking, although other foods may need to be turned only once while cooking. The recipes in this book will suggest when to shake or rearrange the food.

4. Air fry until the food is fully cooked. The recipes will suggest a cooking time, but units may vary slightly. Double-check that the food is cooked until done and is not just golden brown. For meat, you can check the cooking progress by using a meat thermometer inserted into the center of the meat. For vegetables and fruits, pierce the food with a fork or the tip of a knife to determine if it is as tender as desired.

What temperatures should you look for to see if meat or poultry is done? Insert the thermometer into the thickest portion of the meat, not touching fat or bone. The internal temperature should reach at least the following levels:

- 160°F. Hamburgers, sausages, and other ground meats
- 165°F. All poultry
- 145°F. Pork, lamb, veal or beef, chops, steaks, roasts and other whole cuts or meat, and fish.

After cooking, all meat should rest at least 3 minutes. The rest time will allow the internal temperature to climb and the juices to redistribute for better taste.

Tips for Best Performance

Cut the food into uniformly sized pieces for even cooking. Smaller pieces will cook faster than larger ones. Spread the food in an even, thin layer in the air fryer basket.

Do you need to preheat the air fryer? Some manufacturers recommend preheating and others do not. For the recipes in this book, only the recipes that require preheating will say so. If you preheat, or if you are cooking a second batch of food in a hot air fryer, the cooking time may be 1–2 minutes less than the time listed in the recipe.

A light mist of oil is all that is needed when cooking with an air fryer. Recipes will often say to spray the food for 1 or 2 seconds with nonstick cooking spray. As an alternative, use an oil mister to lightly spray the food. Choose oils such as olive oil or canola oil, and avoid oils with saturated fats.

Cleaning an air fryer is generally quite easy. The air fryer basket and tray or drawer under the air fryer basket should be cleaned after each use. Follow the manufacturer's directions. Some will suggest that the parts are to be washed in hot, soapy water and not placed in the dishwasher, and most recommend avoiding abrasive cleansers.

You can use the air fryer to reheat foods—especially those with a crispy crust that you wish to keep crispy.

Air fryers now have many accessories that are available for the various units. Select only those accessories that are recommended by the manufacturer for your unit. You may find that many of the accessories enable the air fryer to cook a wider variety of foods. Some manufacturers now offer meat racks to make it even easier to cook steaks, chops, or fish fillets. Others offer a baking pan so you can cook casseroles or other combinations of food.

Do not stack items on top of the air fryer or around the edges, as the air fryer will be hot during cooking and air will be circulating. Place the air fryer on a heat-proof board. Note that many countertop manufacturers recommend that people avoid operating hot appliances on granite, quartz, or other countertops.

Selecting an Air Fryer

The air fryer market has grown quickly, with many new sizes, shapes, and models now available. It is wise to do a little research before shopping for an air fryer. Most models are known for quick, hot cooking, and have a wide range of temperature settings.

Currently, there is not a standard size for air fryers, and many models list volume in liters or quarts, which can make it hard for people to visualize how much food they hold. Instead of relying on the volume on the package when selecting an air fryer, visualize what you might want to cook and how large an air fryer basket you think you'll need to cook for your family. If, for example, you want to cook fish fillets, chicken breasts, or other larger pieces of food for a family of four, you might want a larger air fryer basket or even one with a large rack. If you prefer to air fry vegetables, or typically want to cook just one or two servings, a model with a smaller basket would be ideal.

Some units are now listed as "air fry ovens," and that often means they have a rack over a tray instead of a basket. It may mean that you can select an air fry setting or use other oven settings, such as "bake" or "toast." Read the instructions in the manual carefully and don't assume that all models offer the same features. The recipes in this book will work in an air fry oven; just know that you may need to tweak the times and temperatures a little for your unit.

Appetizers and Snacks

Spicy Vegetable Egg Rolls

SERVES: 4 | SERVING SIZE: 1 EGG ROLL (MADE WITH ¼ CUP FILLING AND 1 EGG ROLL WRAPPER)
PREP TIME: 7 MINUTES | COOK TIME: 8–10 MINUTES

1   cup cabbage slaw mix
2   green onions, white and
     green portion, chopped
¼   cup finely chopped red bell
     pepper
4   tablespoons roasted
     flaxseed

1   teaspoon reduced-sodium
     soy sauce
½   teaspoon red pepper flakes
4   egg roll wrappers, each
     about 6½ inches square
1   large egg white
1   teaspoon water
1   teaspoon cornstarch

1 Preheat the air fryer, with the air fryer basket in place, to 400°F.

2 In a medium bowl, combine the slaw mix, green onions, red bell pepper, flaxseed, soy sauce, and red pepper flakes for the filling.

3 Place about ¼ cup filling on each egg roll wrapper. In a small bowl, whisk together the egg white, water, and cornstarch. Brush some of the egg-white mixture on the edges of the egg roll wrapper. Roll up the egg roll, folding in the sides so that the filling is contained. Brush the egg-white mixture on the outside of each egg roll.

4 Place the egg rolls in the air fryer basket in a single layer. Air fry for 8–10 minutes or until brown and crispy. Serve warm.

CHOICES/EXCHANGES: 1 Starch | 1 Fat
BASIC NUTRITIONAL VALUES: **Calories** 130 | Calories from Fat 40 | **Total Fat** 4.5 g | Saturated Fat 0.4 g | Trans Fat 0.0 g | **Cholesterol** 0 mg | **Sodium** 210 mg | **Potassium** 200 mg | **Total Carbohydrate** 18 g | Dietary Fiber 4 g | Sugars 2 g | **Protein** 5 g | **Phosphorus** 95 mg

Southwestern Egg Rolls

SERVES: 16 | SERVING SIZE: ½ EGG ROLL (MADE WITH 3 TABLESPOONS FILLING AND ½ TORTILLA)
PREP TIME: 15 MINUTES | COOK TIME: 13–15 MINUTES

1 teaspoon canola oil
½ cup chopped red onion
2 cloves garlic, minced
1 medium red bell pepper, diced
1 cup canned reduced-sodium black beans, drained and rinsed
¼ cup reduced-fat shredded cheddar cheese
1 cup frozen corn
1 (4-ounce) can diced green chilies
¼ cup minced fresh cilantro
1½ tablespoons fresh lime juice
1 teaspoon chili powder
8 low-carb, high-fiber, whole-wheat flour tortillas, each about 8 inches in diameter (such as Mission Carb Balance Whole-Wheat Soft Tortillas)
Nonstick cooking spray

1 To make the filling, heat the canola oil in a nonstick medium skillet over medium-high heat. Add the onion and cook, stirring frequently, for 3 minutes. Add the garlic and red pepper and cook an additional 2 minutes, stirring frequently. Remove from the heat. Stir in the black beans, cheese, corn, green chilies, cilantro, lime juice, and chili powder. Gently stir to blend well.

> **TIP**
> Do not crowd the tortilla rolls. Many air fryer baskets can comfortably hold these tortilla rolls, but others cannot. If your air fryer basket is smaller, it is better to cook half of the tortilla rolls, then repeat with the remaining tortilla rolls.

2 Place a tortilla on a clean surface. Place about 6 tablespoons bean and red pepper mixture down one side of the tortilla. Roll the tortilla as tightly as possible but avoid any of the filling spilling out. Repeat with the remaining tortillas. Place the tortilla rolls in a single layer, seam side down, in the fryer basket. Spray the tortilla rolls with nonstick spray for 3 seconds.

3 Set the temperature to 400°F and air fry for 8–10 minutes.

CHOICES/EXCHANGES: 1 Starch | ½ Fat
BASIC NUTRITIONAL VALUES: **Calories** 100 | Calories from Fat 20 | **Total Fat** 2.5 g | Saturated Fat 1.0 g | Trans Fat 0.0 g | **Cholesterol** 0 mg | **Sodium** 210 mg | **Potassium** 160 mg | **Total Carbohydrate** 16 g | Dietary Fiber 9 g | Sugars 2 g | **Protein** 4 g | **Phosphorus** 110 mg

Stuffed Portobello Mushrooms

SERVES: 4 | SERVING SIZE: 1 MUSHROOM | PREP TIME: 10 MINUTES | COOK TIME: 13–15 MINUTES

4   medium (3-ounce) portobello mushrooms, each 3–3½ inches in diameter
1   tablespoon olive oil
1   tablespoon fresh lemon juice
¾   cup chopped roma tomato
¼   cup reduced-fat shredded mozzarella cheese
1   teaspoon Italian seasoning
½   teaspoon garlic powder
2   tablespoons whole-wheat panko bread crumbs
2   tablespoons flaxseed
2   tablespoons shredded Parmesan cheese

1 Remove stems from the mushrooms and discard or save for other use. Use the tip of a teaspoon to scrape the gills gently out of each mushroom.

2 In a small bowl, stir together the olive oil and lemon juice. Brush the lemon juice mixture evenly and lightly over each mushroom, inside and out.

3 In a small bowl, stir together the chopped tomatoes, mozzarella, Italian seasoning, and garlic powder. Set aside.

4 In another small bowl, stir together the panko bread crumbs, flaxseed, and Parmesan cheese. Set aside.

5 Place the mushrooms, stem side down, in the air fryer basket. Set the temperature to 375°F and air fry for 5 minutes.

6 Turn the mushrooms over, stem side up. Carefully spoon the tomato mixture into each mushroom cap. Spoon the crumb mixture over each mushroom. Air fry for an additional 8–10 minutes or until the crumbs are golden brown. Serve warm.

CHOICES/EXCHANGES: 1 Nonstarchy Vegetable | 1½ Fat
BASIC NUTRITIONAL VALUES: **Calories** 120 | Calories from Fat 60 | **Total Fat** 7.0 g | Saturated Fat 1.7 g | Trans Fat 0.0 g | **Cholesterol** 7 mg | **Sodium** 75 mg | **Potassium** 460 mg | **Total Carbohydrate** 9 g | Dietary Fiber 3 g | Sugars 3 g | **Protein** 6 g | **Phosphorus** 170 mg

South-of-the-Border Stuffed Jalapeños

SERVES: 10 | SERVING SIZE: 2 JALAPEÑO HALVES (MADE WITH 3 TABLESPOONS FILLING)
PREP TIME: 15 MINUTES | COOK TIME: 17–20 MINUTES

1 tablespoon olive oil	2 cloves garlic, minced
4 ounces ground chicken	½ teaspoon chili powder
¼ cup chopped onion	½ teaspoon ground cumin
¼ cup chopped red bell pepper	½ teaspoon salt
¼ cup frozen corn	3 tablespoons roasted flaxseed
⅔ cup canned reduced-sodium black beans, drained and rinsed	10 large jalapeños, split lengthwise and seeded

1 Heat the olive oil in a large nonstick skillet over medium-high heat. Add the ground chicken and cook, stirring frequently until the chicken is done. Remove the cooked chicken from the skillet with a slotted spoon. Add the onion, red pepper, and corn to the skillet. Cook, stirring frequently, until the vegetables are just tender, about 3–4 minutes. Add the black beans and garlic and heat through. Stir in the chili powder, cumin, salt, and flaxseed.

2 Spoon a heaping tablespoon of filling evenly into each jalapeño half. Place the filled jalapeño halves, cut side up, in a single layer in the air fryer basket. Set the temperature to 400°F and air fry for 9–11 minutes or until the peppers are cooked through.

TIPS

Do not crowd the jalapeño peppers. Air fry the peppers in batches, as needed. Remove the first batch of peppers and keep warm as you air fry subsequent batches.

Most of the heat in jalapeño peppers is in the veins and seeds. Even if you don't enjoy spicy foods, you may enjoy these delicious, seed-free stuffed peppers. Remember, jalapeño peppers and other hot chile peppers contain oils that can burn your skin, eyes, and other membranes. Wear disposable gloves when cutting the peppers or wash your hands thoroughly in warm soapy water immediately after handling them.

CHOICES/EXCHANGES: ½ Starch | 1 Nonstarchy Vegetable | ½ Fat
BASIC NUTRITIONAL VALUES: Calories 80 | Calories from Fat 35 | **Total Fat** 4.0 g | Saturated Fat 0.6 g | Trans Fat 0.0 g | **Cholesterol** 10 mg | **Sodium** 150 mg | **Potassium** 300 mg | **Total Carbohydrate** 9 g | Dietary Fiber 3 g | Sugars 3 g | **Protein** 4 g | **Phosphorus** 80 mg

Cheesy Kale Chips

SERVES: 6 | SERVING SIZE: ½ CUP | PREP TIME: 8 MINUTES | COOK TIME: 10 MINUTES

1 bunch Tuscan kale, ribs removed, leaves cut into 2-inch pieces (about 3 cups)

2 tablespoons olive oil

¼ teaspoon coarse ground black pepper

1 tablespoon grated Parmesan cheese

1 In a large bowl, toss together the kale, olive oil, and pepper.

2 Place half of the kale into the air fryer basket. Set the temperature to 400°F and air fry for 3 minutes. Shake the air fryer basket. Air fry for an additional 2 minutes or until the kale chips are crisp. Remove the kale chips to a serving platter. Repeat with the remaining kale. Sprinkle the kale chips with the Parmesan cheese. Serve warm or at room temperature.

CHOICES/EXCHANGES: 1 Fat

BASIC NUTRITIONAL VALUES: **Calories** 45 | Calories from Fat 45 | **Total Fat** 5.0 g | Saturated Fat 0.8 g | Trans Fat 0.0 g | **Cholesterol** 0 mg | **Sodium** 15 mg | **Potassium** 40 mg | **Total Carbohydrate** 1 g | Dietary Fiber 0 g | Sugars 0 g | **Protein** 1 g | **Phosphorus** 15 mg

Snacking Time Chickpeas

SERVES: 6 | SERVING SIZE: 2 ½ TABLESPOONS | PREP TIME: 5 MINUTES | COOK TIME: 10–15 MINUTES

1   (15-ounce) can no-salt-added chickpeas (garbanzo beans), drained and rinsed
Nonstick cooking spray
½   teaspoon garlic powder
½   teaspoon dried thyme leaves
¼   teaspoon coarse ground black pepper
⅛   teaspoon cayenne, or to taste

1 Pour the chickpeas into a medium bowl. Using a paper towel, pat the chickpeas dry. Spray the chickpeas with the nonstick cooking spray for 2 seconds and toss to coat the chickpeas evenly. Pour the chickpeas into the basket.

> **TIP**
> Be sure to sprinkle the seasoning over the hot chickpeas so the seasonings adhere.

2 In a small bowl, stir together the garlic powder, thyme leaves, pepper, and cayenne; set aside.

3 Set the temperature to 375°F and air fry for 10–15 minutes, or until the chickpeas are golden brown and crisp, shaking the air fryer basket every 5 minutes. Midway through the cooking, spray the chickpeas with nonstick cooking spray for 1 second.

4 Pour the hot chickpeas into a bowl. Immediately toss the chickpeas with the seasoning. Serve warm, or allow the crisp chickpeas to cool and dry completely, then store in an airtight container at room temperature.

CHOICES/EXCHANGES: 1 Starch
BASIC NUTRITIONAL VALUES: **Calories** 80 | Calories from Fat 15 | **Total Fat** 1.5 g | Saturated Fat 0.2 g | Trans Fat 0.0 g | Cholesterol 0 mg | **Sodium** 0 mg | **Potassium** 140 mg | **Total Carbohydrate** 13 g | Dietary Fiber 4 g | Sugars 2 g | **Protein** 4 g | **Phosphorus** 80 mg

Mediterranean Pita Chips with White Bean Herb Dip

SERVES: 8 | SERVING SIZE: ½ PITA BREAD WITH 2 TABLESPOONS DIP
PREP TIME: 10 MINUTES | COOK TIME: 6–8 MINUTES

2 tablespoons olive oil	2 cloves garlic, halved
1 teaspoon fresh lemon juice	1 tablespoon fresh lemon juice
1 teaspoon dried oregano leaves	1 tablespoon minced fresh rosemary
4 low-fat whole-wheat pita breads	1 tablespoon minced fresh flat-leaf (Italian) parsley
White Bean Herb Dip:	¼ teaspoon coarse ground black pepper
1 (16-ounce) can reduced-sodium Great Northern beans, drained and rinsed	

1 In a small bowl, stir together the olive oil, lemon juice, and oregano leaves. Lightly brush the mixture over both sides of each pita bread. Cut each pita bread into 8 even triangles.

2 Place half of the pita triangles in the air fryer basket. Set the temperature to 375°F and air fry for 2 minutes. Shake the air fryer basket. Air fry for an additional 1–2 minutes or until chips are golden and crisp. Set the first batch aside and repeat with the remaining pita triangles.

3 While the pita chips are air frying, make the dip. In the work bowl of a food processor, combine the beans, garlic, lemon juice, rosemary, parsley, and pepper. Process until smooth.

4 Serve the warm pita chips with the bean dip.

CHOICES/EXCHANGES: 1½ Starch | ½ Fat
BASIC NUTRITIONAL VALUES: **Calories** 150 | Calories from Fat 40 | **Total Fat** 4.5 g | Saturated Fat 0.6 g | Trans Fat 0.0 g | **Cholesterol** 0 mg | **Sodium** 210 mg | **Potassium** 190 mg | **Total Carbohydrate** 23 g | Dietary Fiber 5 g | Sugars 0 g | **Protein** 6 g | **Phosphorus** 105 mg

Stuffed Potato Skins

SERVES: 8 | SERVING SIZE: ½ OF A WHOLE POTATO SKIN
PREP TIME: 7 MINUTES PLUS 10 MINUTES COOLING TIME | COOK TIME: 37 MINUTES

2 teaspoons olive oil, divided	¼ cup canned no-salt-added
4 small (3-ounce) red potatoes	black beans, drained and rinsed
1 teaspoon chili powder	¼ cup reduced-fat shredded
¼ teaspoon hot sauce	cheddar cheese
¼ cup finely chopped tomato	2 tablespoons fat-free sour cream
1 green onion, white and green	½ cup chopped, peeled, pitted
portion, chopped	avocado
	1 tablespoon minced fresh cilantro

1 Using 1 teaspoon olive oil, rub the outside of the potatoes. Place the potatoes in the air fryer basket. Set the temperature to 350°F and air fry for 15 minutes. Turn and rearrange the potatoes. Air fry for an additional 15 minutes or until the potatoes are tender and pierce easily with the tip of a sharp knife. Remove the potatoes and set aside for 10 minutes or until they are cool enough to handle.

2 Slice the potatoes in half. Using the tip of a teaspoon, remove the potato from the center of each skin, leaving a thin shell, but taking care to not cut the skin. Reserve the cooked potato for another use.

3 In a small bowl, stir together the remaining olive oil, chili powder, hot sauce, chopped tomato, green onion, and black beans. Spoon the tomato mixture into the center of each potato skin.

4 Place the filled potato skins, cut side up, into the air fryer basket. Set the temperature to 350°F and air fry for 5 minutes. Sprinkle the top of each potato with cheese. Air fry for an additional 2 minutes or until the cheese is melted.

5 Using tongs, carefully lift each potato skin out of the air fryer basket. Garnish the top of each with sour cream, avocado, and cilantro.

CHOICES/EXCHANGES: 1 Starch | ½ Fat
BASIC NUTRITIONAL VALUES: Calories 90 | Calories from Fat 30 | **Total Fat** 3.5 g | Saturated Fat 0.8 g | Trans Fat 0.0 g | **Cholesterol** 4 mg | **Sodium** 50 mg | **Potassium** 220 mg | **Total Carbohydrate** 13 g | Dietary Fiber 3 g | Sugars 1 g | **Protein** 3 g | **Phosphorus** 60 mg

Brussels Sprouts and Cauliflower with Malt Vinegar Aioli

SERVES: 6 | SERVING SIZE: ½ CUP VEGETABLES AND 2 TABLESPOONS DIP
PREP TIME: 15 MINUTES | COOK TIME: 15–20 MINUTES

2 cups medium Brussels sprouts, halved

2 cups bite-size cauliflower florets

⅓ cup all-purpose flour

1 cup whole-wheat panko bread crumbs

½ teaspoon coarse ground black pepper

½ teaspoon garlic powder

⅛ teaspoon salt

3 large egg whites

Nonstick cooking spray

Malt Vinegar Aioli:

⅓ cup fat-free mayonnaise

1 clove garlic, minced

2 tablespoons malt vinegar

2 tablespoons minced fresh flat-leaf (Italian) parsley

CHOICES/EXCHANGES: 1 Starch | 1 Nonstarchy Vegetable | ½ Fat
BASIC NUTRITIONAL VALUES: **Calories** 120 | Calories from Fat 20 | **Total Fat** 2.0 g | Saturated Fat 0.3 g | Trans Fat 0.0 g | **Cholesterol** 0 mg | **Sodium** 220 mg | **Potassium** 370 mg | **Total Carbohydrate** 22 g | Dietary Fiber 3 g | Sugars 4 g | **Protein** 6 g | **Phosphorus** 85 mg

1 Place the Brussels sprouts in a medium bowl. Place the cauliflower in another medium bowl. Sprinkle each with about half of the flour and toss to coat evenly. Set the cauliflower aside.

2 In a medium bowl, combine the panko bread crumbs, pepper, garlic powder, and salt.

3 In a small bowl, whisk together the egg whites. Dip each Brussels sprout in egg white and allow the excess to drain back into the bowl. Add the Brussels sprout to the panko bread crumb mixture and coat lightly and evenly. Set the coated Brussels sprout on a wire rack. Repeat with the remaining Brussels sprouts. Place the coated Brussels sprouts in the air fryer basket. Spray the Brussels sprouts with nonstick cooking spray for 2 seconds.

4 Set the temperature to 400°F and air fry for 5 minutes. Shake the air fryer basket. Air fry for an additional 5–7 minutes or until the Brussels sprouts are tender. Remove the Brussels sprouts to a serving platter; set aside and keep warm.

5 Repeat with the cauliflower florets, dipping each in egg white, coating in the panko bread crumbs, and placing on the wire rack. Place the coated cauliflower in the air fryer basket. Spray the cauliflower with nonstick cooking spray for 2 seconds. Set the temperature to 400°F and air fry for 3–4 minutes. Shake the basket. Air fry for an additional 2–4 minutes or until the cauliflower is tender.

6 While the vegetables are air frying, make the aioli. In a small bowl mix together the mayonnaise, garlic, vinegar, and parsley. Blend until smooth.

7 Serve the vegetables warm, with the aioli.

Buffalo Cauliflower Bites

SERVES: 4 | SERVING SIZE: ½ CUP | PREP TIME: 8 MINUTES | COOK TIME: 5–8 MINUTES

3 cups bite-size cauliflower florets

1 tablespoon olive oil

¼ teaspoon garlic powder

3 tablespoons whole-wheat panko bread crumbs

2 tablespoons wing sauce

1 In a medium bowl, toss the cauliflower florets with the olive oil, garlic powder, and panko bread crumbs.

2 Place the cauliflower in the air fryer basket. Set the temperature to 400°F and air fry for 3–4 minutes. Shake the basket. Air fry for 2–4 minutes or until the cauliflower is tender and the edges are crisp.

3 Transfer the cauliflower to a serving bowl and toss with the wing sauce. Serve warm.

CHOICES/EXCHANGES: 1 Nonstarchy Vegetable | 1 Fat
BASIC NUTRITIONAL VALUES: Calories 70 | Calories from Fat 35 | **Total Fat** 4.0 g | Saturated Fat 0.6 g | Trans Fat 0.0 g | **Cholesterol** 0 mg | **Sodium** 130 mg | **Potassium** 320 mg | **Total Carbohydrate** 9 g | Dietary Fiber 2 g | Sugars 3 g | **Protein** 3 g | **Phosphorus** 50 mg

Chicken Quesadillas

SERVES: 12 | SERVING SIZE: ⅙ OF QUESADILLA | PREP TIME: 10 MINUTES | COOK TIME: 17 MINUTES

½ medium white onion, sliced
1 medium red or green bell pepper, thinly sliced
1 teaspoon canola oil
1 teaspoon ground cumin
½ teaspoon chili powder
1 cup shredded, cooked chicken breast, fat discarded

4 low-carb, high-fiber, whole-wheat flour tortillas, each about 8 inches in diameter (such as Mission Carb Balance Whole-Wheat Soft Tortillas)
1 medium tomato, diced
¾ cup reduced-fat shredded cheddar cheese

1 Place the onion and pepper in a small bowl. Drizzle with canola oil and stir to coat evenly. Spoon the vegetables into the air fryer basket. Set the temperature to 400°F and air fry for 6 minutes. Stir the mixture. Air fry for an additional 3 minutes or until the vegetables are tender. Remove the vegetables from the air fryer basket and place into a medium bowl. Toss with the cumin and chili powder.

> **TIP**
> This is a great recipe to use when you have leftover chicken. In a pinch, use a rotisserie chicken breast. Cut the meat from the bone, discard the skin, and shred the meat.

2 Scatter the shredded chicken evenly on top of 2 tortillas. Divide the pepper mixture between the two tortillas. Sprinkle an equal amount of tomato on each tortilla; same with the cheese. Top each with a tortilla. Place one filled quesadilla in the air fryer and air fry for 4 minutes. Remove and cut in half and then cut each half into thirds. Repeat with the remaining quesadilla. Serve warm.

CHOICES/EXCHANGES: ½ Starch | 1 Lean Protein
BASIC NUTRITIONAL VALUES: Calories 90 | Calories from Fat 30 | **Total Fat** 3.5 g | Saturated Fat 1.5 g | Trans Fat 0.0 g | **Cholesterol** 15 mg | **Sodium** 170 mg | **Potassium** 140 mg | **Total Carbohydrate** 8 g | Dietary Fiber 6 g | Sugars 1 g | **Protein** 7 g | **Phosphorus** 125 mg

South-of-the-Border Pumpkin Seeds

SERVES: 4 | SERVING SIZE: ¼ CUP
PREP TIME: 40 MINUTES PLUS 20 MINUTES DRYING TIME | COOK TIME: 45 MINUTES

1 cup pumpkin seeds from a medium pumpkin	1¼ teaspoons salt, divided
8 cups water	1½ tablespoons olive oil
	½ teaspoon chili powder

1 Remove as much of the flesh from the pumpkin seeds as you can. Place the seeds in a colander and rinse with cold water until all the flesh is removed. Place about 8 cups water into a medium saucepan and add 1 teaspoon salt. Bring the water to a boil and add the pumpkin seeds. Boil for 10 minutes. Rinse and drain the seeds and spread them on paper towels to dry for at least 20 minutes.

> **TIP**
> It is easier to coat the seeds evenly with the olive oil, chili powder, and salt mix if you place them all in a resealable plastic bag. Using your fingers, massage ingredients to coat the seeds evenly before air frying.

2 Toss the seeds with the olive oil, chili powder, and the remaining ¼ teaspoon salt. Place the seeds in the air fryer basket. Set the temperature to 350°F and air fry for 35 minutes, shaking the basket several times during the frying process. The seeds should be crispy and slightly brown in color. Allow the seeds to cool completely before storing in an airtight container.

CHOICES/EXCHANGES: 1 Carbohydrate | 2 Fat
BASIC NUTRITIONAL VALUES: Calories 170 | Calories from Fat 100 | **Total Fat** 11.0 g | Saturated Fat 1.7 g | Trans Fat 0.0 g | **Cholesterol** 0 mg | **Sodium** 190 mg | **Potassium** 260 mg | **Total Carbohydrate** 15 g | Dietary Fiber 5 g | Sugars 0 g | **Protein** 5 g | **Phosphorus** 25 mg

Herbed Nuts

SERVES: 12 | SERVING SIZE: ¼ CUP | PREP TIME: 5 MINUTES | COOK TIME: 20–25 MINUTES

1 large egg white
1 tablespoon sugar
1½ teaspoons minced fresh oregano leaves
1½ teaspoons minced fresh sage leaves
1½ teaspoons minced fresh thyme leaves
1½ teaspoons minced fresh rosemary leaves

1 teaspoon garlic powder
1 teaspoon sea salt
½ teaspoon coarse ground black pepper
1 cup whole almonds
1 cup walnut pieces
1 cup pecan halves
Nonstick cooking spray

1 In a large mixing bowl, whisk the egg white with the sugar, herbs, garlic powder, salt, and pepper. Stir in the nuts and toss to coat evenly.

2 Place the nuts in the air fryer basket. Spray the nuts with nonstick cooking spray for 1 second. Set the temperature to 300°F and air fry for 20–25 minutes or until the nuts are toasted, shaking the air fryer basket every 5 minutes.

TIPS

Purchase raw, unsalted nuts for this recipe. Feel free to substitute the kinds of nuts you prefer.

Serve the nuts warm or cool. Store the nuts in an airtight container for up to 2 weeks.

Fresh herbs provide the best flavor for this recipe. You can substitute dried herb leaves for the fresh, if desired, using ½ teaspoon dried herb leaves instead of 1½ teaspoons fresh minced herbs. Crush the dried herb leaves before using to release the flavor.

CHOICES/EXCHANGES: ½ Carbohydrate | 3 ½ Fat
BASIC NUTRITIONAL VALUES: Calories 200 | Calories from Fat 170 | **Total Fat** 19.0 g | Saturated Fat 1.6 g | Trans Fat 0.0 g | **Cholesterol** 0 mg | **Sodium** 190 mg | **Potassium** 170 mg | **Total Carbohydrate** 7 g | Dietary Fiber 3 g | Sugars 2 g | **Protein** 5 g | **Phosphorus** 120 mg

Sweet Potato Nachos

SERVES: 4 | SERVING SIZE: 1 CUP | PREP TIME: 12 MINUTES | COOK TIME: 22 MINUTES

1 medium (9-ounce) sweet potato, not peeled, sliced crosswise in very thin slices about ⅛ inch or less
Nonstick cooking spray
1½ cups frozen stir fry peppers and onion vegetable blend, partially thawed and drained
½ medium jalapeño pepper, split lengthwise and seeded
¼ cup reduced-fat shredded Mexican blend cheese
¼ cup salsa
⅔ cup thinly sliced radishes
4 cherry tomatoes, cut in fourths
½ cup thinly sliced lettuce
2 tablespoons fat-free sour cream
1 tablespoon minced fresh cilantro

1 Place the sweet potato slices evenly in the air fryer basket. Spray with nonstick cooking spray for 1 second. Spoon the stir fry vegetables evenly over the potatoes. Place the jalapeño over the vegetables, skin side up. Spray with nonstick cooking spray for 1 second.

2 Set the temperature to 375°F and air fry for 20 minutes or until the potatoes are cooked and are just crisp-tender, not overcooked and soft. Remove the jalapeño pepper and place it in a bowl; cover loosely with a kitchen towel and allow to stand for 5 minutes.

3 Sprinkle the cheese evenly over the vegetables. Air fry for 2 minutes or until the cheese is melted.

4 Using the tip of a sharp knife, remove the browned or charred skin from the jalapeño pepper and chop the pepper finely.

5 Using a spatula, lift the potatoes and vegetables out of the air fry basket and arrange in an even layer on a serving platter. Sprinkle the chopped jalapeño over the vegetables. Top with the salsa, radishes, tomatoes, and lettuce, then dollop with sour cream and sprinkle with cilantro. Serve immediately.

CHOICES/EXCHANGES: ½ Starch | 1 Nonstarchy Vegetable | ½ Fat
BASIC NUTRITIONAL VALUES: Calories 100 | Calories from Fat 20 | **Total Fat** 2.5 g | Saturated Fat 1.0 g | Trans Fat 0.0 g | **Cholesterol** 5 mg | **Sodium** 180 mg | **Potassium** 450 mg | **Total Carbohydrate** 17 g | Dietary Fiber 3 g | Sugars 6 g | **Protein** 4 g | **Phosphorus** 95 mg

Asian Edamame

SERVES: 5 | SERVING SIZE: ABOUT 1 CUP PODS
PREP TIME: 3 MINUTES PLUS 10 MINUTES MARINATING TIME | COOK TIME: 10 MINUTES

2   tablespoons orange juice
1   tablespoon reduced-sodium
    soy sauce
1   tablespoon unseasoned rice
    wine vinegar

2   teaspoons sugar-free
    maple-flavored syrup
2   teaspoons sesame seeds
1   (16-ounce) package frozen,
    whole unshelled edamame

1 In a medium bowl, whisk together the orange juice, soy sauce, vinegar, syrup, and sesame seeds. Stir in the edamame pods and let stand for 10 minutes.

2 Using a slotted spoon, remove the edamame from the marinade and place in the air fryer basket. Set the temperature to 400°F and air fry for 5 minutes. Shake the air fryer basket. Air fry for an additional 5 minutes. Cool slightly, then serve.

TIPS

If using a smaller air fryer basket, it is best to air fry the edamame in two batches.

Are you familiar with eating edamame? The beans are hidden inside a pod, but do not be deterred by that! To enjoy edamame, hold one pod with your fingertips, then slide it across your teeth, leaving the beans in your mouth. Discard the pod.

CHOICES/EXCHANGES: 1 Nonstarchy Vegetable | ½ Fat
BASIC NUTRITIONAL VALUES: Calories 50 | Calories from Fat 20 | **Total Fat** 2.0 g | Saturated Fat 0.3 g | Trans Fat 0.0 g | **Cholesterol** 0 mg | **Sodium** 25 mg | **Potassium** 170 mg | **Total Carbohydrate** 4 g | Dietary Fiber 2 g | Sugars 1 g | **Protein** 5 g | **Phosphorus** 65 mg

Breakfast and Such

Crisp Egg Cups

SERVES: 4 | SERVING SIZE: 1 EGG CUP (MADE WITH 1 SLICE WHOLE-WHEAT BREAD AND 1 EGG)
PREP TIME: 5 MINUTES | COOK TIME: 10–13 MINUTES

Nonstick cooking spray
4   slices reduced-calorie
    whole-wheat bread, toasted
1½ tablespoons reduced-fat
    whipped tub margarine
    (such as I Can't Believe It's
    Not Butter Vegetable Oil
    Spread)

1   (2-ounce) slice lean ham
    (approximately
    8 × 2½ inches), all
    fat discarded
4   large eggs
⅛   teaspoon salt
⅛   teaspoon coarse ground
    black pepper

1 Preheat the air fryer, with the air fryer basket in place, to 375°F.

2 Spray 4 (8-ounce) oven-proof custard cups or ramekins with nonstick cooking spray.

3 Remove the crusts from the bread and discard or save for other use. Spread one side of the bread with the margarine. Place the bread, margarine side down, into a ramekin and press gently to shape the bread to the cup. Repeat three more times. Slice the ham into strips about ½ inch wide. Place the strips in a single layer in the cups. Crack one egg into each cup. Sprinkle with salt and pepper.

4 Place the filled, uncovered custard cups in the air fryer basket. Air fry for 10–13 minutes or until the eggs are softly set or done as desired. Carefully remove the ramekins from the air fryer basket. Using a hot pad, hold the cup carefully and run a knife around the sides to transfer to a plate. If desired, garnish with chopped fresh flat-leaf (Italian) parsley just before serving.

> **TIP**
> Use caution when placing or removing the custard cups or ramekins from the air fryer basket. The air fryer basket and the custard cups are hot.

CHOICES/EXCHANGES: ½ Starch | 1 Medium-Fat Protein | ½ Fat
BASIC NUTRITIONAL VALUES: Calories 140 | Calories from Fat 70 | **Total Fat** 8.0 g | Saturated Fat 2.7 g | Trans Fat 0.0 g |
Cholesterol 195 mg | **Sodium** 410 mg | **Potassium** 135 mg | **Total Carbohydrate** 6 g |
Dietary Fiber 1 g | Sugars 1 g | **Protein** 12 g | **Phosphorus** 150 mg

Sunday Morning French Toast

SERVES: 4 | SERVING SIZE: 2 HALVES FRENCH TOAST, ½ CUP SLICED STRAWBERRIES, 2 TABLESPOONS
FAT-FREE GREEK YOGURT, AND 1½ TEASPOONS ROASTED FLAXSEED
PREP TIME: 5 MINUTES | COOK TIME: 9 MINUTES

4 slices reduced-calorie
   whole-wheat bread
⅔ cup egg substitute
Nonstick cooking spray
2 cups sliced fresh
   strawberries

½ cup plain fat-free Greek
   yogurt
2 tablespoons roasted
   flaxseed

1 Cut each bread slice in half and place in a shallow dish. Pour the egg substitute over the bread slices. Spray the air fry basket with nonstick cooking spray for 3 seconds. Place the bread halves in a single layer in the air fryer basket, allowing the excess egg substitute to drip back into the dish as you're transferring the bread to the basket.

2 Set the temperature to 400°F and air fry for 9 minutes, turning at least twice during cooking time.

3 Serve warm with strawberries and a dollop of yogurt. Sprinkle roasted flaxseed evenly over each serving.

TIP
Flaxseed is a nutritious seed that can be sprinkled on cereal or fruit or used in a variety of dishes. It is now readily sold in grocery stores as whole seeds or ground into a meal or flour. Read the label carefully to see what kind you are purchasing. Whole flaxseed can be purchased "roasted," but if yours is not, spread the seeds on a baking sheet and bake at 350°F for 5–10 minutes or until the seeds are golden. Store flaxseed in the refrigerator or freezer for up to 6 months.

CHOICES/EXCHANGES: ½ Starch | ½ Fruit | 1 Lean Protein | ½ Fat
BASIC NUTRITIONAL VALUES: **Calories** 140 | Calories from Fat 35 | **Total Fat** 4.0 g | Saturated Fat 0.5 g | Trans Fat 0.0 g | **Cholesterol** 0 mg | **Sodium** 135 mg | **Potassium** 280 mg | **Total Carbohydrate** 18 g | Dietary Fiber 5 g | Sugars 6 g | **Protein** 10 g | **Phosphorus** 125 mg

Tex-Mex Egg Burritos

SERVES: 6 | SERVING SIZE: 1 BURRITO | PREP TIME: 15 MINUTES | COOK TIME: 10–15 MINUTES

1 tablespoon canola oil
1 medium red bell pepper, diced
2 green onions, white and green portion, thinly sliced
4 large eggs
1 (4-ounce) can whole green chilies, drained and coarsely chopped
½ cup diced tomato

6 low-carb, high-fiber, whole-wheat flour tortillas, each about 8 inches in diameter (such as Mission Carb Balance Whole-Wheat Soft Tortillas), warmed
2 ounces reduced-fat shredded cheddar cheese
1 tablespoon salsa

1 Heat the canola oil in a medium skillet over medium-high heat. Add the red pepper and cook for 3 minutes, stirring frequently. Add the green onions and continue to cook, stirring frequently, for 1–2 minutes. Add the eggs and cook until soft set. Stir in the chilies and the tomato.

2 Divide the mixture evenly among the 6 tortillas. Divide the cheese and salsa among the tortillas. Wrap each tortilla as a burrito. Place 3 burritos in the air fryer basket. Set the temperature to 400°F and air fry for 3–5 minutes or until the cheese is melted. Repeat with the remaining burritos. Serve warm.

CHOICES/EXCHANGES: 1 Starch | 1 Nonstarchy Vegetable | 1 Medium-Fat Protein | 1 Fat
BASIC NUTRITIONAL VALUES: Calories 230 | Calories from Fat 100 | **Total Fat** 11.0 g | Saturated Fat 3.9 g | Trans Fat 0.0 g | **Cholesterol** 130 mg | **Sodium** 470 mg | **Potassium** 280 mg | **Total Carbohydrate** 23 g | Dietary Fiber 16 g | Sugars 3 g | **Protein** 12 g | **Phosphorus** 280 mg

Fruit-Studded Granola

SERVES: 18 | SERVING SIZE: ¼ CUP | PREP TIME: 10 MINUTES | COOK TIME: 25–27 MINUTES

1½ cups old-fashioned rolled oats
1 cup pecan halves
1 cup sliced almonds
⅓ cup unsalted pumpkin seeds
⅓ cup unsalted sunflower seeds
¼ cup almond butter
2 tablespoons canola oil
1 tablespoon granulated sucralose sweetener (such as Splenda Blend for Baking)
½ teaspoon almond extract
½ cup chopped dried fruit

1 In a large bowl, mix together the oats, pecans, almonds, pumpkin seeds, and sunflower seeds.

2 In a small, microwave-safe glass bowl, stir together the almond butter, canola oil, and sweetener. Microwave on high (100%) power for 20 seconds. Stir to blend well. Stir in the almond extract. Pour the almond butter mixture over the oats and nut mixture. Stir to coat evenly.

3 Place the granola into the air fryer basket. Set the temperature to 325°F and air fry for 25–27 minutes, or until the granola is golden and crisp, shaking the air fryer basket every 5 minutes. Pour the granola into a large bowl. Allow to cool. Stir in the dried fruit.

TIPS

Serve granola as a snack or sprinkle it on top of fruit or fat-free yogurt. Store the granola, tightly covered, for up to 2–3 weeks. For longer storage, up to about 6 months, tightly cover the granola and store in the freezer.

Choose the dried fruit you enjoy the most. You can purchase a bag of mixed, chopped fruit or select a fruit or two, such as dried apples, berries, or cherries, and chop them. Other choices might include raisins, cranberries, or, for a change of pace, dried pineapple or mango.

Some air fryer baskets or racks have large holes to allow for air circulation. If the holes in your air fryer basket are larger so the oats or nuts may fall through, line the bottom of the basket with parchment paper or place the oat and nut mixture in an ovenproof bowl or baking dish, and place it in the air fryer basket. Check the fit of the bowl or pan before assembling the recipe, and use caution when removing the bowl. Allow the bowl and granola to cool slightly before attempting to remove the filled bowl from the air fryer basket.

CHOICES/EXCHANGES: ½ Starch | ½ Carbohydrate | 2 ½ Fat
BASIC NUTRITIONAL VALUES: Calories 170 | Calories from Fat 120 | **Total Fat** 13.0 g | Saturated Fat 1.2 g | Trans Fat 0.0 g | **Cholesterol** 0 mg | **Sodium** 0 mg | **Potassium** 180 mg | **Total Carbohydrate** 12 g | Dietary Fiber 3 g | Sugars 4 g | **Protein** 4 g | **Phosphorus** 140 mg

Southern Chicken and Waffles

SERVES: 4 | SERVING SIZE: 1 WAFFLE, 4 OUNCES CHICKEN, AND 2 TABLESPOONS SUGAR-FREE SYRUP
PREP TIME: 12 MINUTES | COOK TIME: 15–17 MINUTES

⅓ cup whole-wheat panko bread crumbs

¼ cup chopped pecans

2 tablespoons flaxseed

⅛ teaspoon salt

¼ teaspoon coarse ground black pepper

1 large egg white

1 pound boneless, skinless chicken breasts, all fat discarded, cut into strips about 1 x 2 inches

Nonstick cooking spray

4 frozen reduced-calorie, whole-grain waffles, each about 4 inches in diameter (such as Van's Whole Grain Lite Original Waffles)

½ cup sugar-free maple-flavored syrup

CHOICES/EXCHANGES: 1 ½ Starch | 4 Lean Protein | ½ Fat
BASIC NUTRITIONAL VALUES: **Calories** 310 | Calories from Fat 110 | **Total Fat** 12.0 g | Saturated Fat 1.7 g | Trans Fat 0.0 g | **Cholesterol** 65 mg | **Sodium** 330 mg | **Potassium** 360 mg | **Total Carbohydrate** 25 g | Dietary Fiber 5 g | Sugars 4 g | **Protein** 30 g | **Phosphorus** 350 mg

1 In a shallow bowl, stir together the panko bread crumbs, pecans, flaxseed, salt, and pepper.

2 In another shallow bowl, whisk the egg white until frothy.

3 Dip each chicken piece into the egg white, allowing the excess to drip back into the bowl. Roll the chicken piece in the pecan mixture, coating evenly but lightly. Set the coated chicken piece on a wire rack. Repeat with the remaining chicken pieces.

TIP
Do not crowd the chicken pieces. Many air fryer baskets can comfortably hold these chicken pieces, but others cannot. If your air fryer basket is smaller, it is better to cook half of the chicken pieces, then repeat with the remaining chicken pieces.

4 Place the coated chicken pieces in the air fryer basket. Spray the chicken with nonstick cooking spray for 2 seconds. Set the temperature to 375°F and air fry for 6 minutes. Turn the chicken pieces. Air fry for an additional 5–7 minutes or until the chicken is done and registers 165°F on a meat thermometer. Remove the chicken from the air fryer basket; set aside and keep warm.

5 Place 2 of the waffles in the air fryer basket, separating the waffles into a single layer as much as possible. Spray for 2 seconds with nonstick cooking spray. Set the temperature to 375°F and air fry for 2 minutes or until the waffles are hot and crisp. Repeat with the remaining 2 waffles.

6 To serve, place each waffle on a serving plate, and put an equal amount of chicken on each waffle. Drizzle each serving with 2 tablespoons sugar-free syrup. Serve warm.

Herbed Baked Eggs

SERVES: 2 | SERVING SIZE: 1 EGG
PREP TIME: 2 MINUTES PLUS 1–2 MINUTES STANDING TIME | COOK TIME: 6–7 MINUTES

Nonstick cooking spray
2   large eggs
1   tablespoon soft goat
    cheese crumbles
⅛   teaspoon salt

¼   teaspoon coarse ground
    black pepper
2   teaspoons minced fresh
    flat-leaf (Italian) parsley

1 Spray 2 (8-ounce) oven-proof custard cups or ramekins with nonstick cooking spray.

2 Crack an egg into each ramekin. Top each egg with 1½ teaspoons goat cheese crumbles, then season with salt and pepper. Spray each egg with nonstick cooking spray for 1 second.

3 Place the filled, uncovered custard cups in the air fryer basket. Set the temperature to 350°F and air fry for 6–7 minutes or until the eggs are softly set. Sprinkle the parsley over the eggs. Allow the eggs to stand for 1–2 minutes before serving.

TIPS
Substitute your favorite herb, such as chives, tarragon, or basil, for the parsley.

Do not overcook the eggs, as they will continue to cook and set up after they are removed from the air fryer. Remove them from the air fryer when just softly set.

CHOICES/EXCHANGES: 1 Medium-Fat Protein | ½ Fat
BASIC NUTRITIONAL VALUES: **Calories** 90 | Calories from Fat 50 | **Total Fat** 6.0 g | Saturated Fat 2.1 g | Trans Fat 0.0 g | **Cholesterol** 190 mg | **Sodium** 230 mg | **Potassium** 75 mg | **Total Carbohydrate** 1 g | Dietary Fiber 0 g | Sugars 0 g | **Protein** 7 g | **Phosphorus** 110 mg

Brown Sugar Flaxseed Broiled Grapefruit

SERVES: 2 | SERVING SIZE: ½ GRAPEFRUIT (MADE WITH 1 TEASPOON BROWN SUGAR AND 1 TEASPOON FLAXSEED) | **PREP TIME:** 3 MINUTES | **COOK TIME:** 4 MINUTES

1   small red grapefruit
2   teaspoons granular erythritol sweetener (such as Swerve Brown Sugar replacement)
2   teaspoons flaxseed

1 Preheat the air fryer, with the air fryer basket in place, to 400°F.

2 Cut the grapefruit in half (not through the stem but horizontally). If needed, slice a thin sliver off the bottom of the grapefruit half so it will sit in air fryer basket. Sprinkle each half with 1 teaspoon brown sugar and 1 teaspoon flaxseed.

3 Air fry for 4 minutes. Allow to cool slightly before serving.

> **TIP**
> Some sweeteners, like Swerve Brown Sugar, have a replacement measure of 1:1 for sugar to sweetener. Other brands may recommend a different ratio, so use the amount of sweetener needed to replace 2 teaspoons brown sugar.

CHOICES/EXCHANGES: 1 Fruit
BASIC NUTRITIONAL VALUES: Calories 50 | Calories from Fat 15 | **Total Fat** 1.5 g | Saturated Fat 0.1 g | Trans Fat 0.0 g | **Cholesterol** 0 mg | **Sodium** 0 mg | **Potassium** 170 mg | **Total Carbohydrate** 13 g | Dietary Fiber 2 g | Sugars 7 g | **Protein** 1 g | **Phosphorus** 30 mg

Fish and Seafood

Salmon Sliders with Fennel Slaw

SERVES: 6 | SERVING SIZE: 1 SLIDER (MADE WITH 1 WHOLE-WHEAT SLIDER BUN, 2 OUNCES SALMON, AND ABOUT ½ CUP SLAW) | PREP TIME: 18 MINUTES | COOK TIME: 10 MINUTES

1   medium fennel bulb, cored and sliced very thin

1   medium orange, cut between the membranes into segments

2   tablespoons chopped fresh dill

1   tablespoon fresh lemon juice

1   tablespoon olive oil

¼   teaspoon kosher salt

2   tablespoons roasted flaxseed

¾   pound salmon fillet, cut into 1-inch pieces

¼   cup flat-leaf (Italian) parsley leaves

1   green onion, white and green portion, cut into small pieces

1   teaspoon grated lemon zest

2   tablespoons whole-wheat panko bread crumbs

1   large egg white

Nonstick cooking spray

6   (1-ounce) whole-wheat slider buns, split and toasted

CHOICES/EXCHANGES: 1 Starch | 1 Nonstarchy Vegetable | 2 Lean Protein | 1 Fat

BASIC NUTRITIONAL VALUES: Calories 240 | Calories from Fat 90 | **Total Fat** 10.0 g | Saturated Fat 1.6 g | Trans Fat 0.0 g | **Cholesterol** 30 mg | **Sodium** 300 mg | **Potassium** 540 mg | **Total Carbohydrate** 23 g | Dietary Fiber 5 g | Sugars 6 g | **Protein** 16 g | **Phosphorus** 260 mg

1 In a medium bowl, combine the fennel, orange, dill, lemon juice, olive oil, salt, and flaxseed to make the slaw. Toss gently to mix and set aside.

2 In the work bowl of a food processor, combine the salmon, parsley, green onion, lemon zest, panko bread crumbs, and egg white. Pulse until finely chopped. Remove from the bowl and form into 6 patties about ½ inch thick.

3 Spray one side of each patty with nonstick cooking spray for 3 seconds. Place the patties, sprayed side down, in the air fryer basket. Set the temperature to 400°F and air fry for 5 minutes. Turn the patties over and continue to air fry an additional 5 minutes.

4 Place a salmon patty on each bun half. Top each with about ½ cup slaw and the top bun. Serve immediately.

TIP
Flaxseed is readily sold in grocery stores as whole seeds or ground into a meal or flour. Read the label carefully to see what kind you are purchasing. Whole flaxseed can be purchased "roasted," but if yours is not, spread the seeds on a baking sheet and bake at 350°F for 5–10 minutes or until the seeds are golden. Store flaxseed in the refrigerator or freezer for up to 6 months.

Teriyaki-Glazed Salmon

SERVES: 4 | SERVING SIZE: 3 OUNCES SALMON AND 1½ TABLESPOONS SAUCE
PREP TIME: 5 MINUTES | COOK TIME: 16–17 MINUTES

2 tablespoons reduced-sodium soy sauce
2 tablespoons orange juice
1 tablespoon unseasoned rice vinegar
1 tablespoon honey

2 cloves garlic, minced
2 teaspoons minced ginger
Nonstick cooking spray
4 (4-ounce) salmon fillets, patted dry
1 teaspoon sesame seeds

1 In a small saucepan, over medium-high heat, cook the soy sauce, orange juice, vinegar, honey, garlic, and ginger for 3–4 minutes, stirring frequently. Remove from the heat and set aside.

2 Spray the air fryer basket with nonstick cooking spray for 1 second. Place the salmon fillets in a single layer in the air fryer basket. Spray the top of the salmon with nonstick cooking spray for 2 seconds. Set the temperature to 400°F and air fry salmon for 6 minutes.

3 Brush 2 tablespoons soy–orange mixture over the top of the fish. Air fry fish for an additional 5 minutes. Sprinkle with the sesame seeds. Air fry an additional 2 minutes or until the fish is done and flakes easily with a fork.

4 Serve the fish drizzled with the remaining sauce.

CHOICES/EXCHANGES: ½ Carbohydrate | 3 Lean Protein | 1 Fat
BASIC NUTRITIONAL VALUES: **Calories** 210 | Calories from Fat 80 | **Total Fat** 9.0 g | Saturated Fat 1.9 g | Trans Fat 0.0 g | **Cholesterol** 60 mg | **Sodium** 350 mg | **Potassium** 450 mg | **Total Carbohydrate** 7 g | Dietary Fiber 0 g | Sugars 5 g | **Protein** 23 g | **Phosphorus** 310 mg

Family Favorite Fish Sticks

SERVES: 4 | SERVING SIZE: 4 STICKS | PREP TIME: 8 MINUTES | COOK TIME: 11 MINUTES

1   large egg white
2   tablespoons water
2   tablespoons all-purpose flour
1   cup whole-wheat panko
     bread crumbs
½   teaspoon paprika

½   teaspoon salt-free lemon
     pepper
¾   pound cod fillets, patted
     dry and cut into strips
     about 1 inch wide and
     3 inches long
Nonstick cooking spray

1 In a shallow dish, combine the egg white and water and beat until foamy. In another shallow dish, combine the flour, panko bread crumbs, paprika, and lemon pepper.

2 Dip each fish piece in the egg-white mixture, allowing the excess to drip back into the dish, and then coat with panko mixture. Place the coated fish on a wire rack. Repeat with the remaining fish pieces.

TIP
Do not crowd the fish sticks. Many air fryer baskets can comfortably hold this recipe, but others cannot. If your air fryer basket is smaller, it is better to cook half of the fish sticks, then repeat with the remaining fish sticks.

3 Place the fish sticks in a single layer in the air fryer basket and spray with nonstick cooking spray for 2 seconds. Set the temperature to 400°F and air fry for 5 minutes. Gently turn the fish over. Air fry for an additional 6 minutes or until it is done and crisp.

CHOICES/EXCHANGES: 1 Starch | 2 Lean Protein
BASIC NUTRITIONAL VALUES: **Calories** 150 | Calories from Fat 15 | **Total Fat** 1.5 g | Saturated Fat 0.2 g | Trans Fat 0.0 g | **Cholesterol** 35 mg | **Sodium** 85 mg | **Potassium** 220 mg | **Total Carbohydrate** 15 g | Dietary Fiber 2 g | Sugars 1 g | **Protein** 19 g | **Phosphorus** 125 mg

Fish Tacos with Cilantro Slaw

SERVES: 4 | SERVING SIZE: 1 TACO (MADE WITH 2 OUNCES FISH, 1 TORTILLA, AND ⅓ CUP SLAW)
PREP TIME: 12 MINUTES | COOK TIME: 9–10 MINUTES

8   ounces cod fillets, patted dry
2   teaspoons olive oil, divided
½   teaspoon chili powder
¼   teaspoon ground cumin
¼   teaspoon garlic powder
Nonstick cooking spray
2½ tablespoons fresh lime juice, divided
1¼ cups thinly sliced green cabbage

1   small carrot, shredded
2   tablespoons minced fresh cilantro
4   low-carb, high-fiber, whole-wheat flour tortillas, each about 8 inches in diameter (such as Mission Carb Balance Whole-Wheat Soft Tortillas), warmed

1 Drizzle the fish with 1 teaspoon olive oil, turning to coat evenly.

2 Stir together the chili powder, cumin, and garlic powder. Measure out and set aside ¼ teaspoon seasoning mixture. Sprinkle the remaining seasoning over the fish, coating both sides evenly.

3 Spray the air fryer basket with nonstick cooking spray for 1 second. Place the fish in a single layer in the air fryer basket. Set the temperature to 375°F and air fry for 5 minutes. Turn the fish and air fry for 4–5 minutes or until the fish is done and flakes easily with a fork. Place the fish on a plate and drizzle with 1 tablespoon lime juice. Shred the fish using 2 forks.

4 In a bowl, combine the cabbage, carrot, and cilantro for the slaw. Stir together the remaining 1 teaspoon olive oil, remaining 1½ tablespoons lime juice, and the reserved ¼ teaspoon seasoning mixture. Stir the dressing into the cabbage.

5 To serve, divide the fish among the tortillas. Top each with about ⅓ cup slaw.

CHOICES/EXCHANGES: 1 Starch | 1 Nonstarchy Vegetable | 2 Lean Protein | ½ Fat
BASIC NUTRITIONAL VALUES: **Calories** 200 | Calories from Fat 50 | **Total Fat** 6.0 g | Saturated Fat 1.9 g | Trans Fat 0.0 g | **Cholesterol** 25 mg | **Sodium** 350 mg | **Potassium** 310 mg | **Total Carbohydrate** 23 g | Dietary Fiber 16 g | Sugars 2 g | **Protein** 16 g | **Phosphorus** 220 mg

Tuna Melts

SERVES: 2 | SERVING SIZE: 1 MELT (MADE WITH 1 ENGLISH MUFFIN, 2 ¼ OUNCES TUNA, AND ABOUT ⅔ CUP SALAD) | PREP TIME: 5 MINUTES | COOK TIME: 9 MINUTES

1 (4.5-ounce) can low-sodium chunk light tuna in water, drained
3 teaspoons olive oil, divided
1½ teaspoons balsamic vinegar
1 clove garlic, minced
1 medium stalk celery, chopped

1 green onion, white and green portion, chopped
1 tablespoon minced fresh basil
3 tablespoons sliced almonds
¼ cup reduced-fat shredded cheddar cheese
2 whole-wheat English muffins, split

1 In a medium bowl, stir together the tuna, 1½ teaspoons olive oil, vinegar, garlic, celery, green onion, basil, almonds, and cheese. Set aside.

2 Brush the cut side of the English muffins with the remaining 1½ teaspoons olive oil. Place the muffins, cut side up, in a single layer in the air fryer basket. Set the temperature to 400°F and air fry for 4 minutes or until the muffins are golden and toasted.

3 Carefully spoon the tuna mixture on each muffin, mounding slightly. Air fry for 5 minutes or until the tuna is hot and cheese is melted.

4 Use a flexible, flat spatula to carefully lift each tuna-topped muffin out of the air fryer basket. Serve warm.

CHOICES/EXCHANGES: 2 Starch | 3 Lean Protein | 2 Fat
BASIC NUTRITIONAL VALUES: **Calories** 370 | Calories from Fat 150 | **Total Fat** 17.0 g | Saturated Fat 3.5 g | Trans Fat 0.0 g | **Cholesterol** 35 mg | **Sodium** 470 mg | **Potassium** 430 mg | **Total Carbohydrate** 27 g | Dietary Fiber 5 g | Sugars 2 g | **Protein** 26 g | **Phosphorus** 415 mg

Coconut Shrimp

SERVES: 4 | SERVING SIZE: 4 OUNCES SHRIMP | PREP TIME: 12 MINUTES | COOK TIME: 6–8 MINUTES

1 pound peeled and deveined raw large shrimp (21/30 count)
2 large egg whites, beaten
1 tablespoon water
½ cup whole-wheat panko bread crumbs

¼ cup unsweetened flaked coconut
½ teaspoon ground cumin
½ teaspoon turmeric
½ teaspoon ground coriander
⅛ teaspoon salt
Nonstick cooking spray

1 Pat shrimp dry using paper towels. Place the egg whites and water in a shallow bowl, whisking to combine. Combine the panko bread crumbs, coconut, cumin, turmeric, coriander, and salt in another shallow bowl.

2 Dip each shrimp in the egg mixture, allowing the excess to drip back into the bowl. Then place shrimp in the panko mixture and coat well. Set the coated shrimp on a wire rack. Repeat with all shrimp.

3 Place the shrimp in a single layer in the air fryer basket. Spray the shrimp with nonstick cooking spray for 2 seconds. Set the temperature to 400°F and air fry for 4 minutes. Turn the shrimp over. Air fry for 2–4 minutes or until shrimp are done. Serve warm.

TIPS

Do not crowd the shrimp. Many air fryer baskets can comfortably hold this recipe, but others cannot. If your air fryer basket is smaller, it is better to cook half of the shrimp, then repeat with the remaining shrimp.

If possible, use fresh (never frozen) shrimp or shrimp that are free of preservatives (for example, shrimp that have not been treated with salt or STPP [sodium tripolyphosphate]).

CHOICES/EXCHANGES: ½ Starch | 3 Lean Protein
BASIC NUTRITIONAL VALUES: Calories 180 | Calories from Fat 40 | **Total Fat** 4.5 g | Saturated Fat 3.0 g | Trans Fat 0.0 g | **Cholesterol** 190 mg | **Sodium** 230 mg | **Potassium** 350 mg | **Total Carbohydrate** 9 g | Dietary Fiber 2 g | Sugars 1 g | **Protein** 28 g | **Phosphorus** 270 mg

Cajun Shrimp

SERVES: 2 | SERVING SIZE: 4 OUNCES SHRIMP | PREP TIME: 8 MINUTES | COOK TIME: 5–7 MINUTES

8 ounces peeled and deveined raw large shrimp ($^{2}\!/_{30}$ count)

1 tablespoon olive oil

1 teaspoon salt-free cajun seasoning

$^{1}\!/_{4}$ teaspoon smoked paprika

$^{1}\!/_{8}$ teaspoon salt

1 Preheat the air fryer, with the air fryer basket in place, to 390°F.

2 In a mixing bowl, combine all of the ingredients, coating the shrimp with the oil and the spices. Place the shrimp in a single layer in the air fryer basket. Air fry for 5–7 minutes or until the shrimp turn pink and are done. Serve immediately.

> **TIP**
> If possible, use fresh (never frozen) shrimp or shrimp that are free of preservatives (for example, shrimp that have not been treated with salt or STPP [sodium tripolyphosphate]).

CHOICES/EXCHANGES: 3 Lean Protein | ½ Fat

BASIC NUTRITIONAL VALUES: Calories 160 | Calories from Fat 60 | **Total Fat** 7.0 g | Saturated Fat 1.0 g | Trans Fat 0.0 g | **Cholesterol** 190 mg | **Sodium** 260 mg | **Potassium** 280 mg | **Total Carbohydrate** 1 g | Dietary Fiber 0 g | Sugars 0 g | **Protein** 24 g | **Phosphorus** 245 mg

Baja Shrimp Tacos

SERVES: 4 | SERVING SIZE: 1 TACO (MADE WITH 1 CORN TORTILLA, 2 TABLESPOONS SALSA, AND 2½ OUNCES SHRIMP)
PREP TIME: 15 MINUTES PLUS 10 MINUTES MARINATING TIME | COOK TIME: 16–17 MINUTES

10 ounces peeled and deveined raw medium shrimp ($^{36}/_{40}$ count)

1 (8-ounce) can sliced pineapple in pineapple juice, drained, reserving juice

1 teaspoon olive oil

¼ teaspoon red pepper flakes

¼ teaspoon ground cumin

1 clove garlic, minced

Nonstick cooking spray

½ medium jalapeño pepper, seeded and minced

2 tablespoons minced fresh cilantro

4 corn tortillas, each about 6 inches in diameter, warmed

1 avocado, peeled, pitted, and sliced

2 radishes, thinly sliced

½ cup thinly sliced iceberg lettuce

1 green onion, white and green portion, thinly sliced

4 cherry tomatoes, chopped

CHOICES/EXCHANGES: 1 Starch | ½ Fruit | 2 Lean Protein | ½ Fat
BASIC NUTRITIONAL VALUES: **Calories** 220 | Calories from Fat 60 | **Total Fat** 7.0 g | Saturated Fat 1.0 g | Trans Fat 0.0 g | **Cholesterol** 120 mg | **Sodium** 80 mg | **Potassium** 510 mg | **Total Carbohydrate** 23 g | Dietary Fiber 5 g | Sugars 7 g | **Protein** 18 g | **Phosphorus** 260 mg

1 Place the shrimp in a small bowl. Pour 2 tablespoons reserved pineapple juice over the shrimp. Add the olive oil, red pepper flakes, cumin, and garlic. Stir well and allow to marinate for 10 minutes.

2 Spray the air fryer basket with nonstick cooking spray for 1 second. Pat the pineapple slices dry. Arrange the pineapple slices in the air fryer basket. Spray the slices with nonstick cooking spray for 1 second.

TIP
If possible, use fresh (never frozen) shrimp or shrimp that are free of preservatives (for example, shrimp that have not been treated with salt or STPP [sodium tripolyphosphate]).

3 Set the temperature to 375°F and air fry pineapple for 12 minutes or until the slices are beginning to brown and caramelize. Remove the pineapple slices and set them aside.

4 Drain the shrimp and pat dry; discard the marinade. Arrange the shrimp in a single layer in the air fryer basket. Air fry for 2 minutes. Shake the air fryer basket and air fry for an additional 2−3 minutes or until the shrimp are done and are beginning to turn pink.

5 When the pineapple is cool enough to handle, chop the pineapple. Stir together the chopped pineapple, jalapeño, and cilantro.

6 To assemble the tacos, divide the shrimp evenly among the tortillas. Top with about 2 tablespoons pineapple salsa, and then with sliced avocado, radishes, lettuce, green onion, and tomatoes.

Greek Shrimp on Salad Greens

SERVES: 4 | SERVING SIZE: 2½ CUPS SALAD (MADE WITH 2 OUNCES SHRIMP AND 2 TABLESPOONS DRESSING)
PREP TIME: 15 MINUTES PLUS 30 MINUTES MARINATING TIME | COOK TIME: 4–5 MINUTES

8 ounces peeled and deveined raw medium shrimp ($36/40$ count)

5 tablespoons fresh lemon juice

4 tablespoons olive oil

3 cloves garlic, minced

1 teaspoon dried oregano leaves

¼ teaspoon red pepper flakes

4 cups torn salad greens (such as Romaine, butter lettuce, or other greens)

1 medium red bell pepper, thinly sliced

½ medium red onion, thinly sliced

¼ medium cucumber, thinly sliced

1 cup canned no-salt-added chickpeas (garbanzo beans), drained

¾ cup sliced white button mushrooms

4 tablespoons fat-free crumbled feta cheese

2 tablespoons minced fresh flat-leaf (Italian) parsley

CHOICES/EXCHANGES: ½ Starch | 2 Nonstarchy Vegetable | 2 Lean Protein | 2 Fat
BASIC NUTRITIONAL VALUES: **Calories** 290 | Calories from Fat 140 | **Total Fat** 15.0 g | Saturated Fat 2.1 g | Trans Fat 0.0 g | **Cholesterol** 95 mg | **Sodium** 135 mg | **Potassium** 580 mg | **Total Carbohydrate** 21 g | Dietary Fiber 6 g | Sugars 6 g | **Protein** 19 g | **Phosphorus** 260 mg

1 Place the shrimp in a bowl.

2 In a small bowl, stir together the lemon juice, olive oil, garlic, oregano leaves, and red pepper flakes. Pour 1½ tablespoons lemon juice mixture over the shrimp. Toss the shrimp to cover evenly. Cover the shrimp and refrigerate for 30 minutes. Set the remaining lemon juice mixture aside.

TIP
If possible, use fresh (never frozen) shrimp or shrimp that are free of preservatives (for example, shrimp that have not been treated with salt or STPP [sodium tripolyphosphate]).

3 Arrange the salad greens on salad plates. Top greens with red bell pepper slices, red onion slices, cucumber slices, chickpeas, and sliced mushrooms. Set aside.

4 Drain the shrimp and pat dry; discard the marinade. Place the shrimp in a single layer in the air fryer basket. Set the temperature to 375°F and air fry for 2 minutes. Shake the air fryer basket. Air fry for an additional 2–3 minutes or until the shrimp are done and are beginning to turn pink.

5 Arrange the hot, cooked shrimp on each salad. Drizzle each salad with reserved lemon juice mixture. Sprinkle with feta cheese and parsley.

Meat and Poultry

Sticky Chicken Bites

SERVES: 4 | SERVING SIZE: 4 OUNCES CHICKEN WITH ABOUT 1 TABLESPOON SAUCE
PREP TIME: 5 MINUTES | COOK TIME: 12–14 MINUTES

1   pound boneless, skinless chicken breasts, all fat discarded, cut into ¾-inch cubes
1   tablespoon cornstarch
½   teaspoon smoked paprika
¼   teaspoon coarse ground black pepper
Nonstick cooking spray

3   tablespoons apricot sugar-free all-fruit spread
2   teaspoons reduced-sodium soy sauce
1   clove garlic, minced
1   teaspoon minced fresh ginger
½   teaspoon hot sauce

1 Pat the chicken cubes dry with a paper towel.

2 In a small bowl, stir together the cornstarch, paprika, and pepper. Sprinkle the cornstarch mixture over the chicken cubes and toss to coat evenly.

3 Place the chicken cubes in the air fryer basket. Spray with nonstick cooking spray for 2 seconds. Set the temperature to 375°F and air fry for 5 minutes. Shake the air fryer basket. Air fry an additional 5–6 minutes or until the chicken is almost done.

4 In a small bowl, stir together the apricot spread, soy sauce, garlic, ginger, and hot sauce. Spoon out and reserve about half of the sauce. Brush the chicken cubes lightly with the remaining sauce. Air fry for 2–3 minutes or until the chicken is done and the edges are golden. A meat thermometer inserted in the center of the cubes should register 165°F. Arrange on a serving plate. Drizzle with the remaining apricot mixture.

CHOICES/EXCHANGES: ½ Fruit | 3 Lean Protein
BASIC NUTRITIONAL VALUES: Calories 170 | Calories from Fat 25 | **Total Fat** 3.0 g | Saturated Fat 0.8 g | Trans Fat 0.0 g | **Cholesterol** 65 mg | **Sodium** 180 mg | Potassium 220 mg | **Total Carbohydrate** 10 g | Dietary Fiber 0 g | Sugars 6 g | **Protein** 24 g | **Phosphorus** 180 mg

Buttermilk Fried Chicken

SERVES: 4 | SERVING SIZE: 4 OUNCES CHICKEN
PREP TIME: 12 MINUTES PLUS 15 MINUTES MARINATING TIME | COOK TIME: 14–17 MINUTES

⅓ cup low-fat buttermilk
¼ teaspoon hot sauce
1 pound boneless, skinless chicken breasts, all fat discarded, cut in half lengthwise
6 tablespoons cornflakes
3 tablespoons stone-ground cornmeal
1 teaspoon garlic powder
1 teaspoon paprika
¼ teaspoon salt
¼ teaspoon coarse ground black pepper
Nonstick cooking spray

1 In a deep bowl, stir together the buttermilk and hot sauce. Place the chicken in the buttermilk mixture. Allow to stand 15 minutes.

2 Place the cornflakes into the work bowl of a food processor. Process until coarse crumbs form. Add the cornmeal, garlic powder, paprika, salt, and pepper and pulse until evenly mixed. Pour the crumbs into a shallow bowl.

3 Drain the chicken, allowing the excess buttermilk to drip back into the bowl. Coat the chicken pieces evenly in the cornflake mixture. Place the coated chicken pieces on a wire rack.

4 Place the chicken in the air fryer basket. Spray with nonstick cooking spray for 2 seconds. Set the temperature to 375°F and air fry for 7 minutes. Turn the chicken pieces. Air fry for an additional 7–10 minutes or until the chicken is done and a meat thermometer inserted in the center registers 165°F.

> **TIPS**
> Do not crowd the chicken. Many air fryer baskets can comfortably hold this chicken, but others cannot. If your air fryer basket is smaller, it is better to cook half of the chicken, then repeat with the remaining chicken.
>
> Buttermilk Fried Chicken is really tasty when served with the Creamy Gravy on page 73.

CHOICES/EXCHANGES: ½ Starch | 3 Lean Protein
BASIC NUTRITIONAL VALUES: **Calories** 160 | Calories from Fat 30 | **Total Fat** 3.5 g | Saturated Fat 0.8 g | Trans Fat 0.0 g | **Cholesterol** 65 mg | **Sodium** 190 mg | **Potassium** 230 mg | **Total Carbohydrate** 7 g | Dietary Fiber 1 g | Sugars 0 g | **Protein** 24 g | **Phosphorus** 185 mg

Herb–Marinated Fried Chicken

SERVES: 4 | SERVING SIZE: 3 OUNCES CHICKEN
PREP TIME: 13 MINUTES PLUS 4–12 HOURS MARINATING TIME | COOK TIME: 14 MINUTES

1   (5.5-ounce) container plain fat-free Greek yogurt
4   green onions, white and green portion, cut into small pieces
1½ cups fresh cilantro leaves
½   cup fresh mint leaves
½   cup fresh flat-leaf (Italian) parsley leaves
1   teaspoon ground cumin
⅛   teaspoon salt
¾   pound boneless, skinless chicken breasts, trimmed of fat, pounded until even and about ¼ inch thick
Nonstick cooking spray

1 To make the marinade, place the yogurt, onions, cilantro, mint, parsley, cumin, and salt into a blender. Blend until smooth.

2 Place the chicken pieces into a resealable plastic bag and pour the yogurt marinade over the chicken pieces. Move the chicken pieces around so that each piece is covered with marinade. Seal the bag and marinate in the refrigerator for 4–12 hours.

3 Spray the air fryer basket with nonstick cooking spray for 2 seconds. Remove the chicken from the marinade and allow excess to drip off; discard the marinade in the bag. There should still be marinade on the chicken. Place the chicken in a single layer in the air fryer basket. Set the temperature to 400°F and air fry for 7 minutes. Turn each piece of chicken. Air fry for an additional 7 minutes or until the chicken is done and a meat thermometer inserted in the center registers 165°F.

CHOICES/EXCHANGES: 3 Lean Protein
BASIC NUTRITIONAL VALUES: **Calories** 120 | Calories from Fat 25 | **Total Fat** 3.0 g | Saturated Fat 0.7 g | Trans Fat 0.0 g | **Cholesterol** 50 mg | **Sodium** 110 mg | **Potassium** 270 mg | **Total Carbohydrate** 3 g | Dietary Fiber 1 g | Sugars 1 g | **Protein** 21 g | **Phosphorus** 180 mg

Popcorn Chicken

SERVES: 4 | SERVING SIZE: 3 OUNCES CHICKEN | PREP TIME: 8 MINUTES | COOK TIME: 8–10 MINUTES

¾ pound boneless, skinless chicken breasts, all fat discarded
1 tablespoon olive oil
5 tablespoons whole-wheat Italian-seasoned bread crumbs

3 tablespoons whole-wheat panko bread crumbs
Nonstick cooking spray

1 Preheat the air fryer, with the air fryer basket in place, to 400°F.

2 Cut the chicken into bite-size pieces. Put the olive oil in a shallow bowl and toss chicken pieces in the olive oil to coat.

3 In another shallow bowl, combine the seasoned bread crumbs and the panko bread crumbs. A few pieces at a time, coat the chicken with the crumb mixture and place on a wire rack.

> **TIP**
> Do not crowd the chicken pieces. Many air fryer baskets can comfortably hold the chicken, but others cannot. If your air fryer basket is smaller, it is better to cook half the chicken and then repeat with the remaining chicken.

4 Place the chicken in a single layer in the air fryer basket, making sure not to crowd the pieces. Lightly spray the chicken with nonstick cooking spray for 2 seconds. Air fry for 5 minutes. Shake the air fryer basket. Air fry an additional 3–5 minutes, or until the chicken is done and a meat thermometer inserted in the center registers 165°F.

CHOICES/EXCHANGES: ½ Starch | 3 Lean Protein
BASIC NUTRITIONAL VALUES: Calories 170 | Calories from Fat 50 | **Total Fat** 6.0 g | Saturated Fat 1.2 g | Trans Fat 0.0 g | **Cholesterol** 50 mg | **Sodium** 200 mg | **Potassium** 170 mg | **Total Carbohydrate** 6 g | Dietary Fiber 1 g | Sugars 1 g | **Protein** 19 g | **Phosphorus** 150 mg

Chicken Satay with Peanut Sauce

SERVES: 4 | SERVING SIZE: 4 OUNCES CHICKEN WITH ABOUT 3 TABLESPOONS SAUCE
PREP TIME: 12 MINUTES PLUS 30 MINUTES MARINATING TIME | COOK TIME: 10–12 MINUTES

20–25 (4–5-inch) wooden
skewers, soaked for
30 minutes
¼ cup light coconut milk
1 teaspoon reduced-sodium
soy sauce
3 cloves garlic, minced
1 tablespoon minced fresh
ginger
1 pound boneless, skinless
chicken breasts, all fat
discarded, cut into thin
strips about ¼ × 3 inches
Nonstick cooking spray

Peanut Sauce:
½ cup reduced-sodium,
reduced-sugar creamy
peanut butter
¼ cup reduced-sodium
chicken broth
1 tablespoon fresh lime juice
2 teaspoons hot sauce (such
as Sriracha)
½ teaspoon granulated
sucralose sweetener (such
as Splenda Blend for
Baking)

Garnish:
2 tablespoons minced fresh
cilantro

CHOICES/EXCHANGES: ½ Carbohydrate | 4 Lean Protein | 2 ½ Fat
BASIC NUTRITIONAL VALUES: **Calories** 320 | Calories from Fat 170 | **Total Fat** 19.0 g | Saturated Fat 3.4 g | Trans Fat 0.0 g | **Cholesterol** 65 mg | **Sodium** 220 mg | **Potassium** 460 mg | **Total Carbohydrate** 8 g | Dietary Fiber 2 g | Sugars 3 g | **Protein** 31 g | **Phosphorus** 280 mg

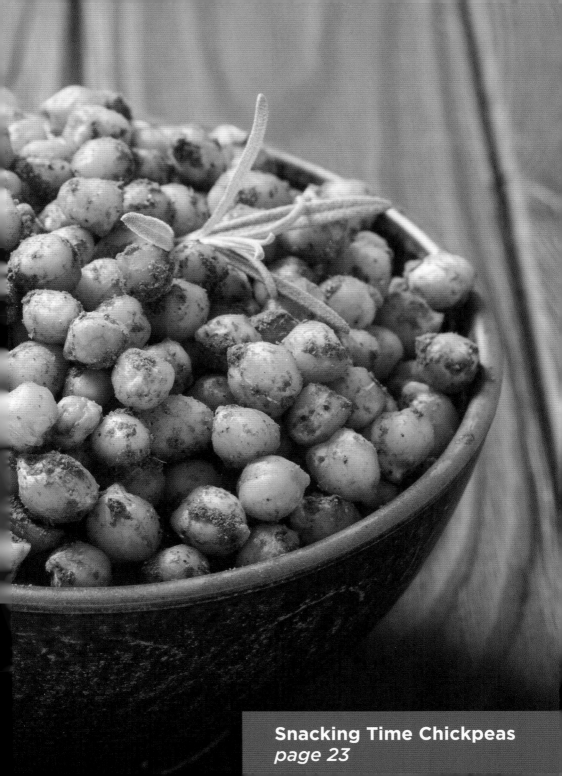

Snacking Time Chickpeas
page 23

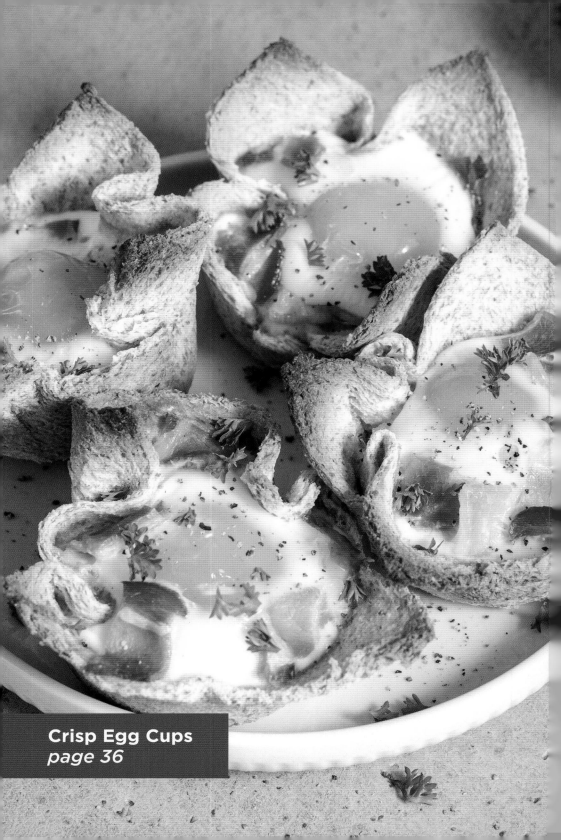

Crisp Egg Cups
page 36

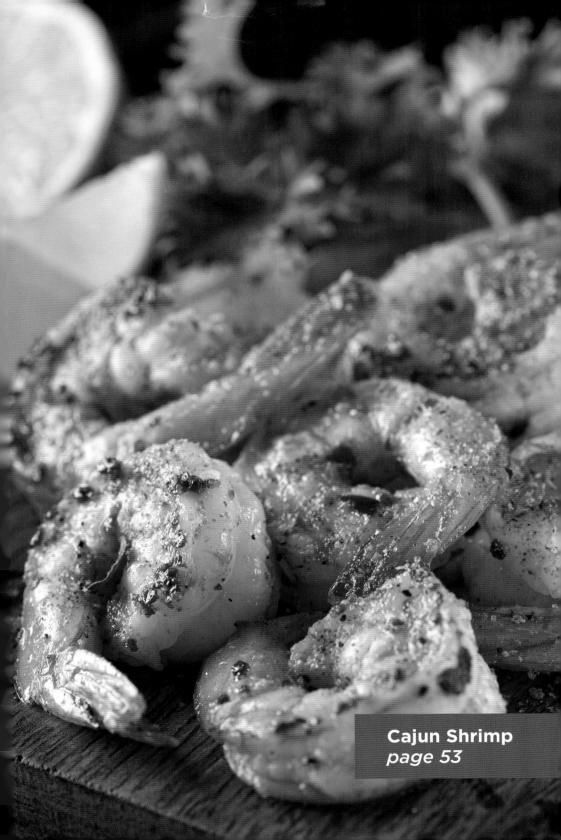

Cajun Shrimp
page 53

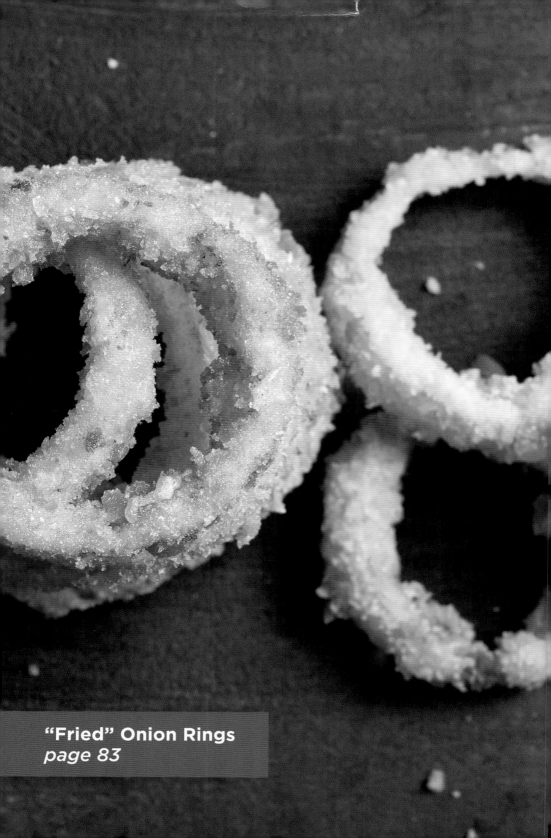

"Fried" Onion Rings
page 83

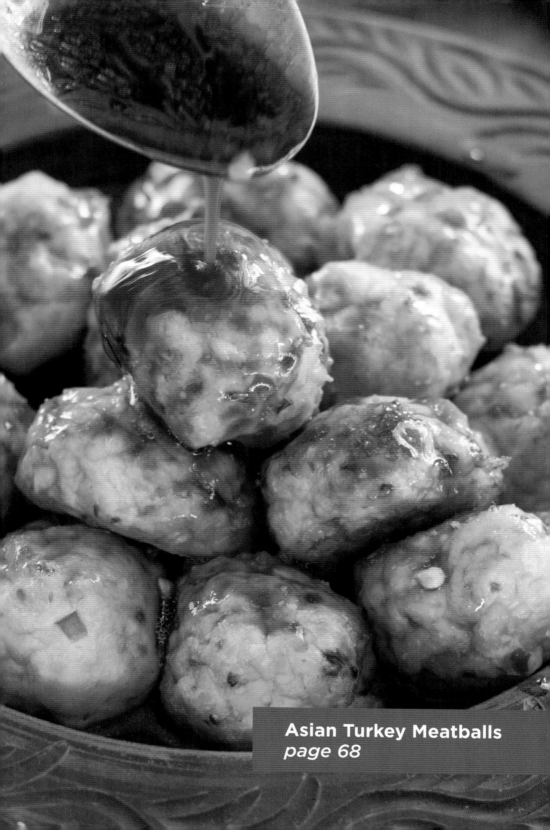

Asian Turkey Meatballs
page 68

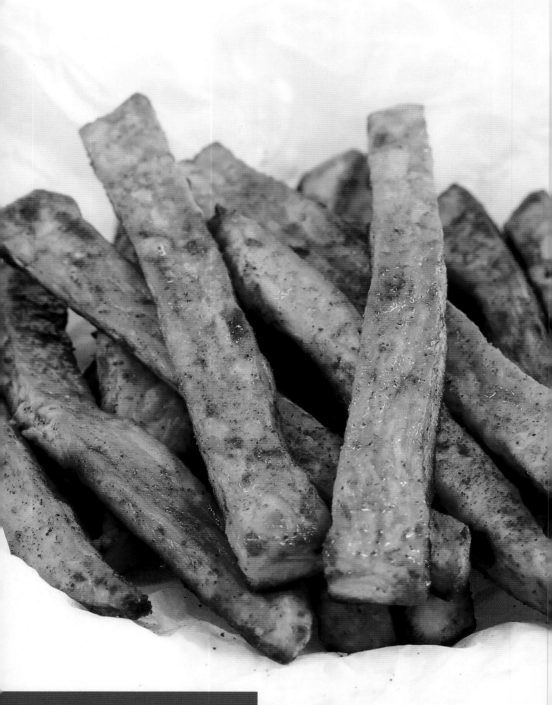

Sweet Potato Fries
page 89

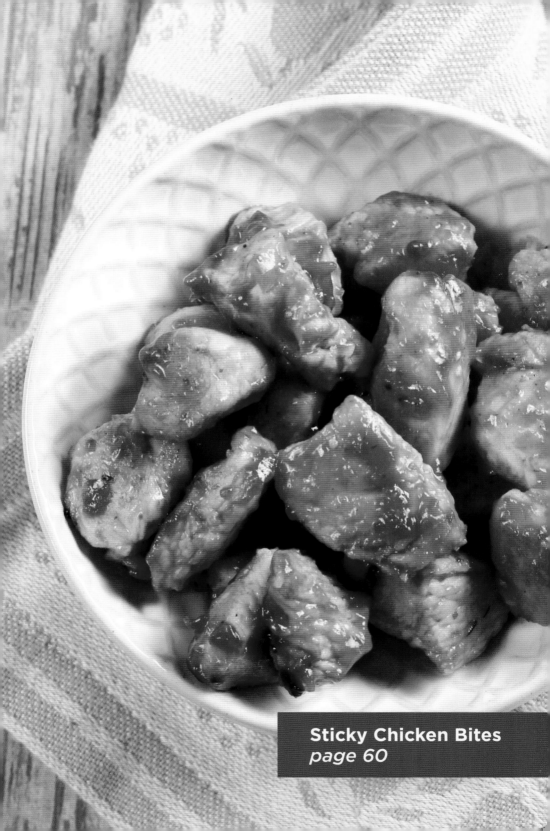

Sticky Chicken Bites
page 60

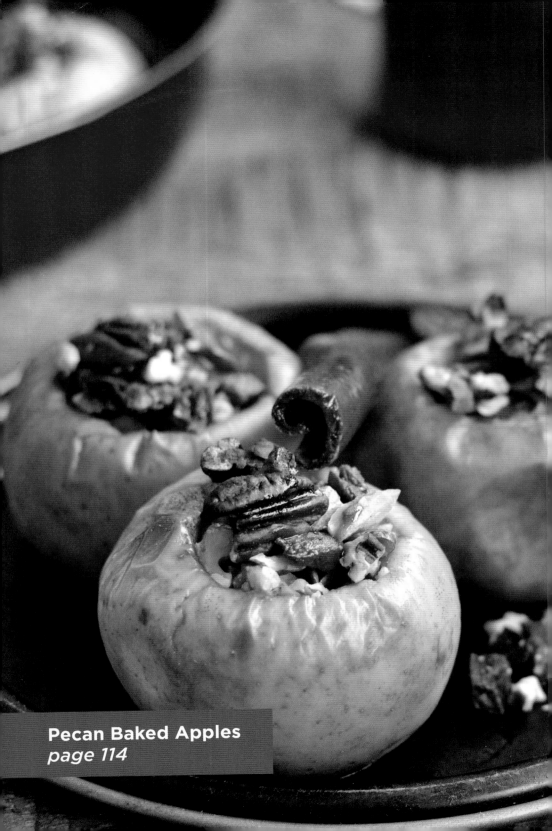

Pecan Baked Apples
page 114

1 Once the wooden skewers have soaked, drain and pat the skewers dry.

2 In a deep bowl, stir together the coconut milk, soy sauce, garlic, and ginger. Add the chicken strips and stir gently to coat the chicken. Cover and refrigerate for 30 minutes.

3 Drain the chicken and discard the marinade. Pat the chicken strips dry with a paper towel. Thread the chicken strips onto the soaked skewers. Place the skewers in a single layer in the air fryer basket. Spray the chicken with nonstick cooking spray for 2 seconds.

TIP
Chicken Satay is often served on skewers. Be sure the skewers you select fit into the air fryer basket, then soak them for 30 minutes in water to cover. If you do not wish to use skewers, you can arrange the chicken in a single layer in the air fryer basket and cook as directed.

4 Set the temperature to 400°F and air fry for 5 minutes. Turn each skewer. Air fry for an additional 5–7 minutes or until the chicken is done and meat thermometer inserted in the center registers 165°F.

5 Meanwhile, in a small, microwave-safe glass bowl, stir together the peanut butter, chicken broth, lime juice, hot sauce, and sweetener. Microwave on high (100%) power for 20 seconds or until the sauce is warm and the peanut butter melts. Stir to blend until smooth.

6 Sprinkle the chicken skewers with the cilantro. Serve the chicken skewers with the peanut sauce.

Open-Faced Chicken Parmesan Sliders

SERVES: 4 | SERVING SIZE: 1 SLIDER (MADE WITH 3 OUNCES CHICKEN, 1½ TABLESPOONS MOZZARELLA, ½ TABLESPOON PARMESAN, AND ½ WHOLE-WHEAT SLIDER BUN)
PREP TIME: 10 MINUTES | COOK TIME: 13–14 MINUTES

1 pound boneless, skinless chicken breast, trimmed of fat, pounded until even and about ¼ inch thick
1 tablespoon olive oil
1 teaspoon Italian seasoning
½ teaspoon garlic powder
½ teaspoon pepper
6 tablespoons whole-wheat panko bread crumbs
4 tablespoons flaxseed
1 medium onion, very thinly sliced

1 medium red or green bell pepper, very thinly sliced
¼ cup reduced-sodium marinara sauce
6 tablespoons part-skim shredded mozzarella cheese
2 tablespoons shredded Parmesan cheese
2 (1-ounce) whole-wheat slider buns, toasted

CHOICES/EXCHANGES: 1½ Starch | 1 Nonstarchy Vegetable | 4 Lean Protein | 1 Fat
BASIC NUTRITIONAL VALUES: Calories 360 | Calories from Fat 130 | **Total Fat** 14.0 g | Saturated Fat 3.1 g | Trans Fat 0.0 g | **Cholesterol** 70 mg | **Sodium** 300 mg | **Potassium** 540 mg | **Total Carbohydrate** 27 g | Dietary Fiber 7 g | Sugars 7 g | **Protein** 33 g | **Phosphorus** 375 mg

1 Cut the chicken breasts into 4 even portions about 3–4 inches square. Lightly brush each side of the chicken pieces with olive oil.

2 In a small bowl, mix together Italian seasoning, garlic powder, and pepper; sprinkle over each side of the chicken pieces, covering evenly.

3 In another small bowl, mix together the panko bread crumbs and the flaxseed. Coat each side of the chicken lightly with the panko bread crumb mixture.

4 Place the chicken in a single layer in the air fryer basket. Set the temperature to 380°F and air fry for 6 minutes. Turn each piece of chicken. Arrange the onion and bell pepper slices over the chicken. Air fry for an additional 6 minutes or until the chicken is done and a meat thermometer inserted in the center registers 165°F.

5 Dollop 1 tablespoon marinara over the vegetables slices on each piece of chicken, then top with 1½ tablespoons mozzarella and ½ tablespoon Parmesan cheese. Air fry for 1–2 minutes or until the cheese is melted.

6 Lift the chicken, topped with the melted cheese and vegetables, out of the air fryer basket and place on one half of a toasted slider bun. Serve warm.

Asian Turkey Meatballs

SERVES: 4 | SERVING SIZE: 5 MEATBALLS WITH ¼ CUP SAUCE
PREP TIME: 15 MINUTES | COOK TIME: 17–20 MINUTES

⅓ cup old-fashioned rolled oats

3 cloves garlic, cut in half

1 green onion, white and green portion, cut into small pieces

1 pound ground turkey breast

1 teaspoon reduced-sodium soy sauce

1 large egg

Nonstick cooking spray

Sweet and Sour Sauce:

2 pitted prunes

1 clove garlic, cut in half

¾ cup reduced-sodium chicken broth

2 tablespoons balsamic vinegar

2 teaspoons reduced-sodium soy sauce

¼ teaspoon granulated sucralose sweetener (such as Splenda Blend for Baking)

¼ teaspoon coarse ground black pepper

1 green onion, white and green portion, chopped

CHOICES/EXCHANGES: ½ Carbohydrate | 4 Lean Protein

BASIC NUTRITIONAL VALUES: Calories 220 | Calories from Fat 40 | **Total Fat** 4.5 g | Saturated Fat 1.2 g | Trans Fat 0.0 g | **Cholesterol** 110 mg | **Sodium** 320 mg | **Potassium** 480 mg | **Total Carbohydrate** 11 g | Dietary Fiber 1 g | Sugars 4 g | **Protein** 32 g | **Phosphorus** 340 mg

1 In the work bowl of a food processor, process the rolled oats until finely chopped. Add 3 cloves garlic and the green onion; pulse until finely chopped.

2 In a large mixing bowl, stir together the turkey, the rolled oat mixture, soy sauce, and the egg. With moistened hands, lightly shape into 20 (1½-inch) meatballs. Arrange the meatballs in a single layer in the air fryer basket. Spray the meatballs with nonstick cooking spray for 2 seconds.

3 Set the temperature to 350°F and air fry for 7 minutes. Turn the meatballs. Air fry an additional 7–9 minutes or until the meatballs are done and a meat thermometer inserted in the center registers 165°F.

4 While the meatballs are air frying, place the prunes and 1 clove garlic in the work bowl of a food processor. Pulse until the prunes are finely chopped. Add the chicken broth and process until well blended and the prunes are very finely chopped. Pour the prune mixture into a small saucepan. Stir in the balsamic vinegar, soy sauce, sweetener, and pepper. Heat over medium heat, stirring frequently, until the mixture comes to a boil. Reduce the heat to low and simmer 1–2 minutes. Remove from the heat.

5 Place the cooked meatballs in a serving bowl. Pour the hot sauce over the meatballs and stir to coat well. Sprinkle with the green onions.

TIPS

If desired, in addition to the green onion, garnish with 1½ teaspoons toasted sesame seeds just before serving.

Do not crowd the meatballs. Many air fryer baskets can comfortably hold these meatballs, but others cannot. If your air fryer basket is smaller, it is better to cook half of the meatballs, then repeat with the remaining meatballs.

Nashville Hot Chicken

SERVES: 4 | SERVING SIZE: 4 OUNCES CHICKEN
PREP TIME: 10 MINUTES PLUS AT LEAST 30 MINUTES MARINATING TIME | COOK TIME: 18–22 MINUTES

1   pound boneless, skinless chicken breasts, all fat discarded, pounded thin
¾   cup low-fat buttermilk
2   tablespoons hot wing sauce

½   cup crushed bran cereal flakes (about 1 cup whole flakes)
1   teaspoon garlic powder
1   teaspoon cayenne pepper
⅛   teaspoon salt
Nonstick cooking spray

1 Slice chicken into strips (about 12 strips total). Combine the buttermilk and hot wing sauce in a shallow dish. Add chicken strips to the mixture and refrigerate for 30 minutes, or up to overnight.

2 In a shallow bowl, stir together the crushed bran cereal, garlic powder, cayenne pepper, and salt.

3 Drain the chicken; discard the marinade in the bowl, shake any excess off the chicken, then dip the chicken strips into the cereal mixture to coat. Place the coated chicken on a wire rack.

4 Place about half the chicken strips in the air fryer basket. Spray the chicken with nonstick cooking spray for 2 seconds. Set the temperature to 375°F and air fry for 5 minutes. Turn the chicken and air fry to 4–6 minutes or until the chicken is done and a meat thermometer inserted in the center registers 165°F.

5 Remove the chicken strips from the air fryer basket and keep warm. Repeat with the second batch of chicken strips.

CHOICES/EXCHANGES: ½ Starch | 3 Lean Protein
BASIC NUTRITIONAL VALUES: Calories 180 | Calories from Fat 35 | **Total Fat** 4.0 g | Saturated Fat 0.9 g | Trans Fat 0.0 g | Cholesterol 65 mg | **Sodium** 260 mg | **Potassium** 290 mg | **Total Carbohydrate** 10 g | Dietary Fiber 2 g | Sugars 2 g | **Protein** 25 g | **Phosphorus** 240 mg

Roasted Turkey and Corn Salad

SERVES: 4 | SERVING SIZE: 2 CUPS SALAD AND 2 OUNCES TURKEY
PREP TIME: 12 MINUTES | COOK TIME: 18 MINUTES

8 ounces boneless, skinless turkey breast, all fat discarded, cut into bite-size pieces
4 teaspoons olive oil, divided
1 teaspoon smoked paprika
1 teaspoon ground cumin
¾ cup frozen corn, partially thawed and drained
Nonstick cooking spray
2 green onions, white and green portion, thinly sliced

1 (16-ounce) can reduced-sodium chickpeas (garbanzo beans), drained and rinsed
1 cup cherry tomatoes, halved
1¼ cups chopped green cabbage
2 tablespoons fresh lemon juice
1 teaspoon white balsamic vinegar
2 tablespoons minced fresh cilantro

1 Place the turkey in a small bowl. Drizzle with 1 teaspoon olive oil, then sprinkle with the paprika and cumin. Toss to coat evenly.

2 Place the turkey in the air fryer basket. Set the temperature to 375°F and air fry for 8 minutes.

3 Stir and turn the turkey. Spread the corn evenly over the turkey. Spray with nonstick cooking spray for 2 seconds. Air fry for 5 minutes; stir and air fry for 5 additional minutes or until the turkey is done and a meat thermometer inserted in the center registers 165°F.

4 Spoon the cooked turkey and corn into a serving bowl. Add the green onions, chickpeas, tomatoes, and cabbage.

5 In a small bowl, stir together the remaining 1 tablespoon olive oil, the lemon juice, and balsamic vinegar. Pour the lemon juice mixture over the turkey mixture. Add the cilantro and toss.

CHOICES/EXCHANGES: 1 ½ Starch | ½ Nonstarchy Vegetable | 2 Lean Protein | ½ Fat
BASIC NUTRITIONAL VALUES: Calories 250 | Calories from Fat 70 | **Total Fat** 8.0 g | Saturated Fat 1.1 g | Trans Fat 0.0 g | **Cholesterol** 25 mg | **Sodium** 125 mg | **Potassium** 520 mg | **Total Carbohydrate** 29 g | Dietary Fiber 7 g | Sugars 7 g | **Protein** 18 g | **Phosphorus** 235 mg

Cracker-Coated Tenderloin

SERVES: 4 | SERVING SIZE: 3 OUNCES PORK | PREP TIME: 10 MINUTES | COOK TIME: 6–7 MINUTES

½   cup low-fat buttermilk
¾   cup crushed no-salt soda
    crackers (about 15 crackers)
½   teaspoon salt-free lemon
    pepper

12   ounces pork tenderloin,
    all visible fat discarded
Nonstick cooking spray

1 Pour the buttermilk into a shallow dish. In another shallow dish, combine the cracker crumbs and lemon pepper.

2 Cut the tenderloin into 4 equal pieces. Pound each slice until very thin (the thinner you pound these, the tastier they will be). Dip each piece in the buttermilk, allowing excess to drip back into the dish, then coat with crumb mixture. Place on a wire rack.

> **TIP**
> Do not crowd the pork pieces. Many air fryer baskets can comfortably hold these pork pieces, but others cannot. If your air fryer basket is smaller, it is better to cook half of the pork, then repeat with the pork.

3 Spray the air fryer basket with nonstick cooking spray for 2 seconds. Spray both sides of the pork with nonstick spray for 3 seconds. Place the pork in the air fryer basket in a single layer. Be sure not to crowd the pork pieces. Set the temperature to 400°F and air fry for 6–7 minutes or until the pork is done and a meat thermometer inserted in the center registers at least 145°F.

CHOICES/EXCHANGES: ½ Starch | 2 Lean Protein
BASIC NUTRITIONAL VALUES: **Calories** 150 | Calories from Fat 35 | **Total Fat** 4.0 g | Saturated Fat 0.9 g | Trans Fat 0.0 g | **Cholesterol** 45 mg | **Sodium** 65 mg | **Potassium** 360 mg | **Total Carbohydrate** 9 g | Dietary Fiber 0 g | Sugars 1 g | **Protein** 18 g | **Phosphorus** 170 mg

Creamy Gravy

Crispy pork tenderloin is often served with creamy, pepper-seasoned gravy. You can capture that old-fashioned flavor today.

SERVES: 4 | SERVING SIZE: 2 TABLESPOONS | PREP TIME: NONE | COOK TIME: ABOUT 5 MINUTES

1 tablespoon reduced-fat stick margarine (such as I Can't Believe It's Not Butter Stick Original, 79% Vegetable Oil Spread)

1½ tablespoons all-purpose flour

¼ teaspoon coarse ground black pepper

⅔ cup skim milk

1 Melt the margarine in a small saucepan over medium–high heat. Stir in the flour and cook for 1 minute, stirring constantly and blending until the mixture is smooth. Season with pepper. Gradually blend in the skim milk. Cook, stirring constantly, until mixture bubbles and thickens.

2 Spoon about 2 tablespoons gravy over each serving.

CHOICES/EXCHANGES: ½ Carbohydrate | ½ Fat
BASIC NUTRITIONAL VALUES: **Calories** 50 | Calories from Fat 25 | **Total Fat** 3.0 g | Saturated Fat 0.9 g | Trans Fat 0.0 g | **Cholesterol** 0 mg | **Sodium** 40 mg | **Potassium** 70 mg | **Total Carbohydrate** 4 g | Dietary Fiber 0 g | Sugars 2 g | **Protein** 2 g | **Phosphorus** 45 mg

Pork with Warm Bean Salad

SERVES: 4 | SERVING SIZE: 2 CUPS SALAD WITH 3 OUNCES PORK
PREP TIME: 10 MINUTES PLUS 3 MINUTES STANDING TIME | COOK TIME: 23 MINUTES

12 ounces pork tenderloin, all fat discarded, cut into slices about ¾ inch thick

2 tablespoons olive oil, divided

1½ teaspoons Italian seasoning, divided

1 small red or sweet yellow onion, halved and thinly sliced

1 medium red bell pepper, cut into strips about ½ inch wide

2 cloves garlic, minced

¼ teaspoon coarse ground black pepper

1 cup sliced button or white mushrooms

1 (15.5-ounce) can reduced-sodium cannellini beans, drained and rinsed

5 cups fresh spinach leaves, stems removed

1 tablespoon fresh lemon juice

CHOICES/EXCHANGES: 1 Starch | 1 Nonstarchy Vegetable | 3 Lean Protein | ½ Fat
BASIC NUTRITIONAL VALUES: **Calories** 270 | Calories from Fat 90 | **Total Fat** 10.0 g | Saturated Fat 1.8 g | Trans Fat 0.0 g | **Cholesterol** 45 mg | **Sodium** 95 mg | **Potassium** 830 mg | **Total Carbohydrate** 23 g | Dietary Fiber 6 g | Sugars 3 g | **Protein** 24 g | **Phosphorus** 285 mg

1 Place the pork slices in a single layer on a plate. Using 2 teaspoons olive oil, lightly brush both sides of the pork. Sprinkle ½ teaspoon Italian seasoning evenly over the pork.

2 Place the onion, red pepper, and garlic in a mixing bowl. Drizzle with 1 tablespoon olive oil; toss to coat the vegetables evenly. Sprinkle with the remaining 1 teaspoon Italian seasoning and the pepper and toss to coat evenly.

3 Place the meat and vegetables in the air fryer basket. Set the temperature to 375°F and air fry for 9 minutes.

4 While the pork is air frying, toss the sliced mushrooms with the remaining 1 teaspoon olive oil in a small bowl.

5 Stir the vegetables and turn the pork in the air fryer basket. Add the mushrooms to the air fryer basket. Air fry for 9 minutes. Stir the vegetables and turn the pork. Pour the beans evenly over the pork. Air fry for an additional 5 minutes or until the beans are warm and the pork is done; a meat thermometer inserted in the center should register at least 145°F. Allow the pork and vegetables to stand and cool for 3 minutes.

6 Arrange the spinach on a platter. Spoon the warm pork and beans over the spinach. Drizzle with the lemon juice. Serve immediately.

Diner-Style Pork Chops

SERVES: 4 | SERVING SIZE: 4 OUNCES PORK
PREP TIME: 10 MINUTES PLUS 5 MINUTES STANDING TIME | COOK TIME: 17–18 MINUTES

4   (4-ounce) boneless center cut pork chops, cut about ¾ inch thick, all fat trimmed and discarded
1   large egg white
2   tablespoons water
3   tablespoons whole-wheat panko bread crumbs
½   teaspoon dried thyme leaves
½   teaspoon dried sage
½   teaspoon coarse ground black pepper
Nonstick cooking spray

1 Pat the pork chops dry.

2 In a shallow bowl, whisk together the egg white and water.

3 In another shallow bowl, combine the panko bread crumbs, thyme, sage, and pepper.

4 Dip each pork chop in the egg-white mixture, turning to coat evenly and allowing the excess to drip back into the bowl. Then quickly dip them in the crumb mixture, turning to coat lightly, but evenly.

> **TIP**
> Do not crowd the chops. Many air fryer baskets can comfortably hold these chops, but others cannot. If your air fryer basket is smaller, it is better to cook half of the chops, then repeat with the remaining chops.

5 Place the chops in the air fryer basket. Spray the chops with nonstick cooking spray for 2 seconds. Set the temperature to 375°F and air fry for 12 minutes. Turn the chops; spray with nonstick cooking spray for 1 second. Air fry an additional 5–6 minutes or until the chops are done and a meat thermometer inserted in the center registers at least 145°F. Allow the chops to stand 5 minutes before serving.

CHOICES/EXCHANGES: 3 Lean Protein | 1 Fat
BASIC NUTRITIONAL VALUES: Calories 180 | Calories from Fat 70 | **Total Fat** 8.0 g | Saturated Fat 2.6 g | Trans Fat 0.0 g | Cholesterol 60 mg | **Sodium** 60 mg | **Potassium** 320 mg | **Total Carbohydrate** 3 g | Dietary Fiber 1 g | Sugars 0 g | **Protein** 22 g | **Phosphorus** 180 mg

Beef Fajitas

SERVES: 4 | SERVING SIZE: 1 FAJITA (MADE WITH 1 TORTILLA, 3 OUNCES BEEF, AND ½ CUP VEGETABLES)
PREP TIME: 12 MINUTES | COOK TIME: 24 MINUTES

12 ounces lean, boneless beef sirloin, cut into thin strips	½ teaspoon coarse ground black pepper
½ cup thinly sliced white onion	4 tablespoons fresh lime juice
1 medium red bell pepper, thinly sliced	2 tablespoons olive oil
1 medium green bell pepper, thinly sliced	4 low-carb, high-fiber, whole-wheat flour tortillas, each about 8 inches in diameter (such as Mission Carb Balance Whole-Wheat Soft Tortillas), warmed
2 cloves garlic, minced	
½ teaspoon chili powder	
1 teaspoon ground cumin	

1 Place the beef in a medium bowl. Place the sliced onions and peppers in another medium bowl.

2 In a small bowl, whisk together the garlic, chili powder, cumin, pepper, lime juice, and olive oil until blended. Pour about half of the mixture over the beef and the remaining half over the vegetables. Stir well to coat the food in each bowl.

3 Place the vegetables in the air fryer basket. Set the temperature to 400°F and air fry for 6 minutes. Stir the mixture. Air fry for an additional 6 minutes or until the vegetables are tender. Remove the vegetables from the air fryer basket and place in a serving bowl. Cover with aluminum foil to keep warm.

4 Add the beef to the air fryer basket and air fry for 6 minutes. Stir the mixture. Air fry for an additional 6 minutes or until beef is browned and done.

5 Divide the vegetables and beef evenly among the tortillas to serve.

CHOICES/EXCHANGES: 1 ½ Starch | 1 Nonstarchy Vegetable | 2 Lean Protein | 2 Fat
BASIC NUTRITIONAL VALUES: **Calories** 310 | Calories from Fat 120 | **Total Fat** 13.0 g | Saturated Fat 3.7 g | Trans Fat 0.1 g | **Cholesterol** 30 mg | **Sodium** 340 mg | **Potassium** 520 mg | **Total Carbohydrate** 26 g | Dietary Fiber 17 g | Sugars 4 g | **Protein** 23 g | **Phosphorus** 305 mg

Texas Beef Kabobs

SERVES: 4 | SERVING SIZE: 4 OUNCES BEEF (ABOUT 5 SKEWERS)
PREP TIME: 15 MINUTES PLUS AT LEAST 4 HOURS MARINATING TIME | COOK TIME: 20 MINUTES

1 pound beef top round, all fat discarded, sliced into thin strips about ¼ × 3 inches
¼ cup salsa
1 teaspoon chili powder
2 cloves garlic
2 tablespoons red wine vinegar
1 tablespoon olive oil
20–25 (4–5-inch) wooden skewers, soaked for 30 minutes

1 Place the meat strips in a deep bowl.

2 In a small bowl, stir together the salsa, chili powder, garlic, and red wine vinegar. Measure out and reserve 2 tablespoons salsa mixture; cover and refrigerate the reserved salsa. Pour the remaining salsa mixture over the beef. Add the olive oil. Stir to coat the beef. Cover and refrigerate at least 4 hours, or up to overnight.

3 Take the reserved salsa mixture out of the refrigerator so it can come to room temperature.

> **TIP**
> Be sure the skewers you select fit into the air fryer basket, then soak them for 30 minutes in water to cover. If you do not wish to use skewers, you can arrange the beef strips in a single layer in the air fryer basket and cook as directed.

4 Drain the beef and discard the marinade. Once the wooden skewers have soaked, drain and pat dry. Loosely thread the meat strips onto the skewers.

5 Arrange about half of the skewers in a single layer in the air fryer basket. Set the temperature to 375°F and air fry for 5 minutes. Turn and rearrange the skewers. Air fry for an additional 5 minutes or until the beef is cooked and a meat thermometer inserted in the center registers at least 145°F. Set the cooked skewers on a plate and cover with aluminum foil to keep warm. Repeat with the remaining skewers. Drizzle kabobs with the reserved salsa mixture before serving.

CHOICES/EXCHANGES: 4 Lean Protein | ½ Fat
BASIC NUTRITIONAL VALUES: Calories 190 | Calories from Fat 80 | **Total Fat** 9.0 g | Saturated Fat 2.0 g | Trans Fat 0.0 g | **Cholesterol** 60 mg | **Sodium** 115 mg | **Potassium** 280 mg | **Total Carbohydrate** 2 g | Dietary Fiber 0 g | Sugars 0 g | **Protein** 24 g | **Phosphorus** 155 mg

Skirt Steak with Peppers and Spicy Gremolata

SERVES: 4 | SERVING SIZE: 3 OUNCES BEEF AND 2 TABLESPOONS GREMOLATA
PREP TIME: 12 MINUTES PLUS 10 MINUTES RESTING TIME | COOK TIME: 16–18 MINUTES

¾ pound beef skirt steak
½ teaspoon salt
½ teaspoon coarse ground pepper
Nonstick cooking spray
1 medium red bell pepper, cut into strips
½ cup sliced almonds, toasted

1¼ cups packed fresh flat-leaf (Italian) parsley
2 teaspoons grated lime zest (from 2 limes)
2 tablespoons fresh lime juice
1 tablespoon olive oil
1 clove garlic, cut in half
1 teaspoon chile paste

1 Pat skirt steak dry with paper towels. Sprinkle the steak with salt and pepper. Spray the air fryer basket with nonstick cooking spray for 2 seconds. Place the red pepper strips in the air fryer basket.

2 Cut the steak in 4 equal pieces that will fit in the basket, and place the steak pieces in the air fryer basket (pieces may overlap.) Set the temperature to 400°F and air fry for 10 minutes. Rearrange the steak, moving the bottom pieces to the top, and continue to air fry for 6–8 minutes or until a meat thermometer inserted in the center of the steak registers 145°F. Do not overcook the steak or it will be tough.

3 While the steak is cooking, prepare the gremolata. In the work bowl of a food processor, combine the almonds, parsley, lime zest, lime juice, olive oil, garlic, and chile paste. Process until smooth.

4 Allow the steak to rest, covered, for 10 minutes. Spread the steak pieces evenly with the gremolata. Slice the steak very thin and place on a platter. Sprinkle peppers around the steak for serving.

CHOICES/EXCHANGES: ½ Carbohydrate | 3 Lean Protein | 2 Fat
BASIC NUTRITIONAL VALUES: Calories 250 | Calories from Fat 150 | **Total Fat** 17.0 g | Saturated Fat 3.5 g | Trans Fat 0.3 g | **Cholesterol** 55 mg | **Sodium** 350 mg | **Potassium** 450 mg | **Total Carbohydrate** 7 g | Dietary Fiber 3 g | Sugars 2 g | **Protein** 21 g | **Phosphorus** 175 mg

Vegetables and Sides

Cauliflower Tots

SERVES: 6 | SERVING SIZE: 3 TOTS | PREP TIME: 12 MINUTES | COOK TIME: 24 MINUTES

½ medium head cauliflower or 4 cups florets
¼ cup reduced-fat shredded cheddar cheese
3 tablespoons grated Parmesan cheese
¼ cup all-purpose flour
1 large egg
Nonstick cooking spray

1 Grate the cauliflower with a box grater or finely chop in a food processor. This should produce about 3 cups grated cauliflower. If the cauliflower seems liquid, place in the center of a clean kitchen towel and squeeze to eliminate moisture.

2 In a large bowl, mix the grated cauliflower with the cheddar cheese, Parmesan cheese, flour, and egg; blend well. Shape the mixture into 18 small "tot" shapes (about 1 tablespoon per tot).

3 Place half of the tots in a single layer in the air fryer basket. Spray the cauliflower tots with nonstick cooking spray for 3 seconds. Set the temperature to 400°F and air fry for 12 minutes. Repeat with the remaining tots. Serve warm.

> **TIP**
> The cauliflower tots can easily be frozen before air frying. Mix and shape tots as directed, then place on a cookie sheet that has been lined with parchment paper. Freeze until firm. Place the frozen tots in a freezer bag, seal, and label. When ready to serve, air fry in the air fryer as directed, adding 1–2 minutes to the air frying time, or as needed, until the tots are browned.

CHOICES/EXCHANGES: 1 Nonstarchy Vegetable | 1 Fat
BASIC NUTRITIONAL VALUES: **Calories** 80 | Calories from Fat 30 | **Total Fat** 3.5 g | Saturated Fat 1.4 g | Trans Fat 0.0 g | **Cholesterol** 35 mg | **Sodium** 100 mg | **Potassium** 210 mg | **Total Carbohydrate** 8 g | Dietary Fiber 1 g | Sugars 1 g | **Protein** 5 g | **Phosphorus** 95 mg

"Fried" Onion Rings

SERVES: 4 | SERVING SIZE: ABOUT 8–10 RINGS | PREP TIME: 16 MINUTES | COOK TIME: 20 MINUTES

1 egg
1 tablespoon water
¾ cup whole-wheat panko bread crumbs
½ teaspoon cajun seasoning

1 medium (10-ounce) sweet onion (such as Vidalia), cut into ¼-inch slices
Nonstick cooking spray

1 Preheat the air fryer, with the air fryer basket in place, to 400°F.

2 Whisk together the egg and water in a shallow bowl for dipping. Place the panko bread crumbs and seasoning in another shallow bowl and combine well. Separate the onion into rings. Dip the rings, one at a time, in the egg mixture, turning to coat but allowing the excess to drip back into the bowl. Dip in panko mixture and coat well. Place on a wire rack. Discard any remaining egg mixture.

3 Place about half of the coated onions in the air fryer basket. Spray with nonstick cooking spray for 2 seconds. Air fry for 10 minutes or until tender and browning on the edges. Repeat with remaining coated onion rings. Keep cooked onion rings warm in the oven until ready to serve.

CHOICES/EXCHANGES: ½ Starch | 1 Nonstarchy Vegetable | ½ Fat
BASIC NUTRITIONAL VALUES: Calories 90 | Calories from Fat 20 | **Total Fat** 2.0 g | Saturated Fat 0.4 g | Trans Fat 0.0 g | **Cholesterol** 30 mg | **Sodium** 70 mg | **Potassium** 120 mg | **Total Carbohydrate** 16 g | Dietary Fiber 2 g | Sugars 4 g | **Protein** 4 g | **Phosphorus** 60 mg

Spicy Green Beans

SERVES: 4 | **SERVING SIZE:** ½ CUP | **PREP TIME:** 10 MINUTES | **COOK TIME:** 9–11 MINUTES

12 ounces green beans, trimmed

1 tablespoon olive oil

1 teaspoon chile garlic paste

1 tablespoon whole-wheat panko bread crumbs

¼ teaspoon salt

1 Place the green beans in a medium bowl and toss with the olive oil, chile garlic paste, panko bread crumbs, and salt.

2 Place the green beans in the air fryer basket. Set the temperature to 400°F and air fry for 4 minutes. Shake the air fryer basket. Air fry for an additional 5–7 minutes. Serve warm.

CHOICES/EXCHANGES: 1 Nonstarchy Vegetable | ½ Fat

BASIC NUTRITIONAL VALUES: **Calories** 60 | Calories from Fat 30 | **Total Fat** 3.5 g | Saturated Fat 0.5 g | Trans Fat 0.0 g | **Cholesterol** 0 mg | **Sodium** 160 mg | **Potassium** 115 mg | **Total Carbohydrate** 7 g | Dietary Fiber 2 g | Sugars 1 g | **Protein** 2 g | **Phosphorus** 25 mg

Mexican Street Corn

SERVES: 4 | SERVING SIZE: 1 EAR OF CORN | PREP TIME: 8 MINUTES | COOK TIME: 10–12 MINUTES

4   medium ears sweet corn, husks removed
1   tablespoon olive oil
¼   cup plain fat-free Greek yogurt
¼   cup fat-free mayonnaise
¼   cup chopped fresh cilantro
1   tablespoon fresh lime juice
1   teaspoon grated lime zest
¼   cup crumbled Cotija cheese

1 Brush the ears of corn with the olive oil. Place the corn in the air fryer basket. Set the temperature to 400°F and air fry for 5 minutes. Turn the corn. Air fry for an additional 5–7 minutes.

2 While the corn is air frying, in a small bowl whisk together the yogurt, mayonnaise, cilantro, lime juice, and lime zest.

3 Using a brush or spoon, spread each ear of corn with the yogurt mixture. Sprinkle with the Cotija cheese.

TIPS

You can substitute ¼ cup grated Parmesan cheese for the Cotija cheese.

Do not crowd the corn. Many air fryer baskets can comfortably hold 4 ears of corn. This is one time, however, if need be, you can stack the ears in the air fryer basket, placing 2 or 3 in one direction and placing the remaining ears cross-wise. The more air flowing around the corn, the better.

CHOICES/EXCHANGES: 1 ½ Starch | 1 ½ Fat
BASIC NUTRITIONAL VALUES: **Calories** 180 | Calories from Fat 70 | **Total Fat** 8.0 g | Saturated Fat 2.1 g | Trans Fat 0.0 g | **Cholesterol** 10 mg | **Sodium** 230 mg | **Potassium** 280 mg | **Total Carbohydrate** 25 g | Dietary Fiber 3 g | Sugars 6 g | **Protein** 7 g | **Phosphorus** 160 mg

Carrots with Harissa Sauce

SERVES: 4 | SERVING SIZE: ½ CUP | PREP TIME: 10 MINUTES | COOK TIME: 20–22 MINUTES

1½ pounds carrots, sliced
    ½ inch thick
1   tablespoon apricot sugar-
    free all-fruit spread

2   teaspoons olive oil
1½ teaspoons harissa
1   teaspoon fresh lemon juice

1 Place the carrots in a medium bowl. In a small bowl, stir together the apricot all-fruit spread, the olive oil, harissa, and lemon juice. Pour the harissa sauce over the carrots and stir to coat the carrots evenly.

2 Place the carrots in the air fryer basket. Set the temperature to 380°F and air fry for 20–22 minutes, or until the carrots are tender, shaking the air fryer basket every 5 minutes.

> **TIP**
> Harissa is a spicy paste that is popular in North African and Middle Eastern cooking. The paste begins with a blend of hot chilies and olive oil, and is typically seasoned with garlic, cumin, and other spices. Many larger grocery stores are beginning to stock jars of the paste, but if you can't find it, you can substitute a chile paste or your favorite hot sauce. As the intensity of the heat will vary with the brand, you may want to experiment a little. This carrot dish is not overly hot, but if you are unsure, reduce the harissa to 1 teaspoon the first time you make it. You may find you enjoy the complex flavor of this paste so much you will find lots of uses for it, such as stirring a spoonful into a soup, stew, chili, or even a marinade for a grilled meat.

CHOICES/EXCHANGES: 3 Nonstarchy Vegetable | ½ Fat
BASIC NUTRITIONAL VALUES: Calories 90 | Calories from Fat 25 | **Total Fat** 3.0 g | Saturated Fat 0.4 g | Trans Fat 0.0 g | **Cholesterol** 0 mg | **Sodium** 115 mg | **Potassium** 510 mg | **Total Carbohydrate** 16 g | Dietary Fiber 5 g | Sugars 8 g | **Protein** 2 g | **Phosphorus** 55 mg

Au Gratin Potatoes

SERVES: 4 | SERVING SIZE: ½ CUP | PREP TIME: 5 MINUTES | COOK TIME: 23–24 MINUTES

4 small red potatoes (about 16 ounces), not peeled, cut into cubes about 1 x ¾ inch

Butter-flavored nonstick cooking spray

¼ teaspoon salt-free seasoning blend

⅛ teaspoon salt

⅓ cup reduced-fat shredded cheddar cheese

2 tablespoons whole-wheat panko bread crumbs

2 tablespoons flaxseed

1 tablespoon shredded Parmesan cheese

1 tablespoon minced chives

1 Place the potato cubes in the air fryer basket. Spray with butter-flavored nonstick cooking spray for 2 seconds. Sprinkle with seasoning blend and salt.

2 Set the temperature to 375°F and air fry for 10 minutes. Shake the air fryer basket. Air fry for an additional 10 minutes. Shake the air fryer basket.

3 In a small bowl, stir together the cheddar cheese, panko bread crumbs, flaxseed, and Parmesan cheese. Sprinkle the cheese mixture over the potatoes. Air fry for 3–4 minutes or until the cheese is melted and the crumbs are toasted. Spoon into a serving bowl. Garnish with the chives.

CHOICES/EXCHANGES: 1½ Starch | 1 Fat
BASIC NUTRITIONAL VALUES: Calories 150 | Calories from Fat 45 | **Total Fat** 5.0 g | Saturated Fat 1.4 g | Trans Fat 0.0 g | **Cholesterol** 5 mg | **Sodium** 170 mg | **Potassium** 560 mg | **Total Carbohydrate** 22 g | Dietary Fiber 3 g | Sugars 2 g | **Protein** 6 g | **Phosphorus** 160 mg

Sesame Asparagus

SERVES: 4 | SERVING SIZE: 5–6 ASPARAGUS SPEARS | PREP TIME: 8 MINUTES | COOK TIME: 20 MINUTES

8 ounces asparagus (about 20–25 spears about ⅜ inch in diameter), trimmed

2 tablespoons fat-free mayonnaise

1 teaspoon unseasoned rice vinegar

½ teaspoon reduced-sodium soy sauce

1 clove garlic, minced

¼ cup whole-wheat panko bread crumbs

2 tablespoons sesame seeds

Nonstick cooking spray

1 Place the asparagus in a single layer on a baking sheet.

2 In a small bowl, stir together the mayonnaise, vinegar, soy sauce, and garlic. Using a pastry brush, brush the mixture evenly over the asparagus, coating it completely.

3 In another small bowl, stir together the panko bread crumbs and sesame seeds. Sprinkle the mixture evenly over the asparagus, turning to coat it evenly.

4 Arrange about half of the asparagus in a single layer in the air fryer basket. Spray the asparagus with nonstick cooking spray for 2 seconds. Set the temperature to 400°F and air fry for 5 minutes. Turn the asparagus. Air fry for an additional 5 minutes or until asparagus is crisp-tender and edges are golden. Set the cooked asparagus on a plate, cover, and keep warm. Repeat with the remaining asparagus.

> **TIP**
> Do not crowd the asparagus. Arrange about half of the asparagus in the air fryer basket in a single layer. If your air fryer is larger, you may be able to cook more than half of the asparagus at once.

CHOICES/EXCHANGES: 1 Nonstarchy Vegetable | ½ Fat

BASIC NUTRITIONAL VALUES: Calories 60 | Calories from Fat 25 | **Total Fat** 3.0 g | Saturated Fat 0.4 g | Trans Fat 0.0 g | **Cholesterol** 0 mg | **Sodium** 95 mg | **Potassium** 140 mg | **Total Carbohydrate** 8 g | Dietary Fiber 2 g | Sugars 1 g | **Protein** 3 g | **Phosphorus** 65 mg

Sweet Potato Fries

SERVES: 3 | SERVING SIZE: ABOUT ½–¾ CUP | PREP TIME: 8 MINUTES | COOK TIME: 15–17 MINUTES

½ teaspoon garlic powder
½ teaspoon smoked paprika
¼ teaspoon salt
¼ teaspoon coarse ground
    black pepper

2 medium (9–10-ounce)
    sweet potatoes, not peeled,
    cut into thin sticks about
    ¼ × ¼ × 3 inches
Nonstick cooking spray

1 In a small bowl, stir together the garlic powder, paprika, salt, and pepper; set aside.

2 Put the sweet potato sticks in the air fryer basket, stacking loosely. Spray with nonstick cooking spray for 1 second. Set the temperature to 400°F and air fry for 15–17 minutes, or until the potatoes are cooked and the edges are crisp and brown. Shake the air fryer basket every 5 minutes, and spray midway through cooking with nonstick cooking spray for 1 second. Immediately sprinkle the hot fries with the seasoning mixture.

CHOICES/EXCHANGES: 2 Starch
BASIC NUTRITIONAL VALUES: Calories 140 | Calories from Fat 10 | **Total Fat** 1.0 g | Saturated Fat 0.1 g | Trans Fat 0.0 g | **Cholesterol** 0 mg | **Sodium** 250 mg | **Potassium** 710 mg | **Total Carbohydrate** 31 g | Dietary Fiber 5 g | Sugars 10 g | **Protein** 3 g | **Phosphorus** 80 mg

Crunchy Zucchini Sticks

SERVES: 4 | SERVING SIZE: ½ CUP | PREP TIME: 10 MINUTES | COOK TIME: 14–16 MINUTES

2 large egg whites
¼ teaspoon hot pepper sauce
¼ cup stone-ground cornmeal
½ cup whole-wheat panko bread crumbs
1 teaspoon chili powder
½ teaspoon garlic powder

1 small (10-ounce) zucchini, not peeled, cut into sticks about ⅜ × ⅜ × 2½ inches
Nonstick cooking spray
2 tablespoons crumbled Cotija cheese

1 In a shallow bowl, whisk together the egg whites and hot pepper sauce.

2 In a small bowl, stir together the cornmeal, panko bread crumbs, chili powder, and garlic powder.

3 Dip the zucchini sticks into the egg white, allowing the excess to drip back into the bowl. Roll the zucchini sticks in the crumb mixture, then place on a wire rack.

4 Arrange the zucchini sticks in a single layer in the air fryer basket. Spray with nonstick cooking spray for 2 seconds. Set the temperature to 400°F and air fry for 8 minutes. Shake the basket. Air fry for an additional 6–8 minutes or until the zucchini is brown and crisp. Immediately sprinkle with Cotija cheese.

CHOICES/EXCHANGES: 1 Starch | ½ Fat
BASIC NUTRITIONAL VALUES: Calories 90 | Calories from Fat 20 | **Total Fat** 2.0 g | Saturated Fat 0.8 g | Trans Fat 0.0 g | **Cholesterol** 0 mg | **Sodium** 90 mg | **Potassium** 230 mg | **Total Carbohydrate** 14 g | Dietary Fiber 2 g | Sugars 2 g | **Protein** 4 g | **Phosphorus** 80 mg

Sage-Seasoned Winter Squash

SERVES: 4 | SERVING SIZE: ½ CUP | PREP TIME: 10 MINUTES | COOK TIME: 20 MINUTES

4   cups peeled butternut
    squash cubes, cut into
    about 1-inch cubes
2   tablespoons olive oil
1   teaspoon dry sage leaves
2   cloves garlic, minced

¼   teaspoon salt
¼   teaspoon coarse ground
    black pepper
¼   cup sliced almonds,
    chopped

1 In a large bowl, toss together the squash and the olive oil.

2 In a small bowl, stir together the sage leaves, garlic, salt, and pepper. Sprinkle the seasoning mixture over the squash and toss to coat evenly. Place the squash in the air fryer basket.

3 Set the temperature to 375°F and air fry for 15 minutes. Shake the air fryer basket, then sprinkle the squash with the chopped almonds. Air fry an additional 5 minutes.

CHOICES/EXCHANGES: 1 Starch | 2 Fat
BASIC NUTRITIONAL VALUES: **Calories** 160 | Calories from Fat 90 | **Total Fat** 10.0 g | Saturated Fat 1.2 g | Trans Fat 0.0 g | **Cholesterol** 0 mg | **Sodium** 150 mg | Potassium 550 mg | **Total Carbohydrate** 18 g | Dietary Fiber 4 g | Sugars 3 g | **Protein** 3 g | **Phosphorus** 80 mg

Roasted Butternut Squash Salad

SERVES: 4 | SERVING SIZE: 1 SLICE SQUASH, 2 CUPS LETTUCE, ½ TABLESPOON WALNUTS, AND 2 TABLESPOONS DRESSING | PREP TIME: 7 MINUTES | COOK TIME: 18–20 MINUTES

1 pound butternut squash, peeled and sliced crosswise into 4 slices, each about ¾ inch thick
3 tablespoons olive oil, divided
3 tablespoons finely chopped shallots
2 tablespoons white wine vinegar
1 teaspoon Dijon mustard
1 teaspoon sugar-free maple-flavored breakfast syrup
¼ teaspoon salt
¼ teaspoon coarse ground black pepper
8 cups torn salad greens (such as Romaine, butter lettuce, or other greens)
2 tablespoons chopped walnuts, toasted
1 tablespoon minced fresh sage

1 Lightly brush each side of the squash slices with olive oil, using 1 tablespoon olive oil. Reserve the remaining 2 tablespoons oil.

2 Place the squash slices in a single layer in the air fryer basket. Set the temperature to 375°F and air fry for 10 minutes. Turn and rearrange the slices and air fry an additional 8–10 minutes or until the squash is golden brown and tender.

> **TIP**
> When selecting the squash, choose one that has an elongated neck. You can cut full, pretty slices from the neck for this salad, and reserve the rounded end of the squash for another use.

3 For the dressing, whisk together the shallots, white wine vinegar, Dijon mustard, syrup, salt, and pepper in a small bowl. While whisking, drizzle in the remaining 2 tablespoons olive oil.

4 Arrange the lettuce leaves on individual salad plates. Place a slice of squash on each plate. Drizzle with dressing, then sprinkle with walnuts and fresh sage.

CHOICES/EXCHANGES: ½ Starch | 2½ Fat
BASIC NUTRITIONAL VALUES: **Calories** 150 | Calories from Fat 120 | **Total Fat** 13.0 g | Saturated Fat 1.7 g | Trans Fat 0.0 g | **Cholesterol** 0 mg | **Sodium** 180 mg | **Potassium** 300 mg | **Total Carbohydrate** 10 g | Dietary Fiber 3 g | Sugars 2 g | **Protein** 2 g | **Phosphorus** 45 mg

Crisp Parmesan Broccoli Florets

SERVES: 6 | SERVING SIZE: ½ CUP | PREP TIME: 8 MINUTES | COOK TIME: 10–14 MINUTES

4 cups bite-size broccoli florets
2 tablespoons olive oil
1 teaspoon Italian seasoning
½ teaspoon garlic powder
¼ teaspoon salt
2 tablespoons grated Parmesan cheese

1 In a large bowl, toss the broccoli with the olive oil, Italian seasoning, garlic powder, and salt.

2 Place the broccoli in the air fryer basket. Set the temperature to 400°F and air fry for 5 minutes. Shake the air fryer basket. Air fry for an additional 5–9 minutes or until the broccoli is tender and browned. Place on a serving platter or in a serving bowl. Immediately after air frying and while the broccoli is still hot, sprinkle with the Parmesan cheese.

> **TIP**
> Do not crowd the broccoli. Many air fryer baskets can comfortably hold 3 cups of broccoli florets. If your air fryer basket is smaller, it is better to cook half of the broccoli, then repeat with the remaining broccoli.

CHOICES/EXCHANGES: 1 Nonstarchy Vegetable | 1 Fat

BASIC NUTRITIONAL VALUES: Calories 60 | Calories from Fat 45 | **Total Fat** 5.0 g | Saturated Fat 0.9 g | Trans Fat 0.0 g | **Cholesterol** 0 mg | **Sodium** 130 mg | **Potassium** 160 mg | **Total Carbohydrate** 3 g | Dietary Fiber 1 g | Sugars 1 g | **Protein** 2 g | **Phosphorus** 45 mg

New Potatoes and Green Beans with Vinaigrette

SERVES: 4 | SERVING SIZE: ½ CUP | PREP TIME: 12 MINUTES | COOK TIME: 20–22 MINUTES

12 ounces green beans, trimmed	2 tablespoons apple cider vinegar
6 ounces red potatoes, not peeled, cut into 1-inch cubes	1 tablespoon Dijon mustard
1 tablespoon canola oil	1 tablespoon olive oil
	¼ teaspoon coarse ground black pepper

1 In a large bowl, toss together the green beans, potatoes, and canola oil until the vegetables are evenly coated.

2 Place the potatoes and green beans in the air fryer basket. Set the temperature to 400°F and air fry for 10 minutes. Shake the air fryer basket. Air fry for an additional 10–12 minutes or until the vegetables are tender.

3 While the vegetables are air frying, whisk together the vinegar, mustard, olive oil, and black pepper in a small bowl.

4 Place the green beans and potatoes into a serving bowl and toss with the vinaigrette.

CHOICES/EXCHANGES: ½ Starch | 1 Nonstarchy Vegetable | 1 ½ Fat
BASIC NUTRITIONAL VALUES: **Calories** 120 | Calories from Fat 60 | **Total Fat** 7.0 g | Saturated Fat 0.8 g | Trans Fat 0.0 g | Cholesterol 0 mg | **Sodium** 100 mg | **Potassium** 360 mg | **Total Carbohydrate** 13 g | Dietary Fiber 3 g | Sugars 3 g | **Protein** 2 g | **Phosphorus** 55 mg

Mustard-Glazed Carrots

SERVES: 4 | SERVING SIZE: ½ CUP | PREP TIME: 8 MINUTES | COOK TIME: 14–16 MINUTES

6 carrots (about 1 pound), peeled and sliced ¼ inch thick
1 tablespoon olive oil
1 tablespoon whole-grain mustard
1 tablespoon white wine vinegar
1 shallot, finely chopped
⅛ teaspoon salt
¼ teaspoon coarse ground pepper

1 Toss the carrots in the olive oil. Place the carrots in the air fryer basket. Set the temperature to 400°F and air fry for 14–16 minutes or until done as desired.

> **TIP**
> These carrots are also good served chilled, as a salad.

2 Meanwhile, in a small bowl, whisk together the mustard, vinegar, shallot, salt, and pepper. Toss the mustard mixture with the cooked carrots. Serve warm.

CHOICES/EXCHANGES: 2 Nonstarchy Vegetable | 1 Fat
BASIC NUTRITIONAL VALUES: **Calories** 80 | Calories from Fat 35 | **Total Fat** 4.0 g | Saturated Fat 0.5 g | Trans Fat 0.0 g | **Cholesterol** 0 mg | **Sodium** 200 mg | **Potassium** 350 mg | **Total Carbohydrate** 11 g | Dietary Fiber 3 g | Sugars 5 g | **Protein** 1 g | **Phosphorus** 45 mg

Fried Fennel Rings

SERVES: 4 | SERVING SIZE: ½ CUP | PREP TIME: 8 MINUTES | COOK TIME: 18–25 MINUTES

2   fennel bulbs (each about 8 ounces after trimming), cut horizontally into ⅓-inch slices

1   tablespoon olive oil

⅛   teaspoon salt

1   teaspoon grated lemon zest

3   tablespoons shredded Parmesan cheese

1   Brush fennel slices with olive oil. Place the fennel slices in the air fryer basket, arranging in a single layer, if possible. If not, you may place a second layer on top.

2   In a small bowl, combine the salt and lemon zest, and sprinkle over fennel.

3   Set the temperature to 400°F and air fry for 15–20 minutes or until the fennel is tender. Sprinkle with the Parmesan cheese and continue to air fry for 3–5 minutes or until the cheese is melted and starting to brown. Serve warm.

CHOICES/EXCHANGES: 2 Nonstarchy Vegetable | ½ Fat

BASIC NUTRITIONAL VALUES: Calories 70 | Calories from Fat 35 | **Total Fat** 4.0 g | Saturated Fat 0.8 g | Trans Fat 0.0 g | **Cholesterol** 0 mg | **Sodium** 160 mg | **Potassium** 490 mg | **Total Carbohydrate** 9 g | Dietary Fiber 4 g | Sugars 2 g | **Protein** 2 g | **Phosphorus** 70 mg

Farmer's Market Vegetable Medley

SERVES: 4 | SERVING SIZE: ¾ CUP | PREP TIME: 15 MINUTES | COOK TIME: 25 MINUTES

8   ounces green beans, trimmed

1   medium carrot, halved lengthwise and cut into ¾-inch pieces

½   medium red bell pepper, cut into strips about ½ inch thick

½   medium zucchini, not peeled, halved lengthwise and cut into ¾-inch pieces

¼   medium red onion, halved and thinly sliced

1   tablespoon olive oil

2½   teaspoons reduced-sodium soy sauce

½   teaspoon garlic powder

½   teaspoon dried basil leaves

¼   teaspoon coarse ground black pepper

2   tablespoons minced fresh flat-leaf (Italian) parsley

1 In a mixing bowl, stir together the green beans, carrots, red pepper, zucchini, and onion. Drizzle with the olive oil and soy sauce, and toss to coat well. Sprinkle with the garlic powder, dried basil leaves, and pepper, and toss to coat evenly.

2 Place the vegetables in the air fryer basket. Set the temperature to 375°F and air fry for 15 minutes. Stir the vegetables. Air fry for an additional 10 minutes or until vegetables are crisp-tender. Sprinkle with the minced parsley just before serving.

> **TIP**
> This recipe is a great way to cook fresh vegetables from your own garden or the local market. If desired, substitute a green pepper for the red pepper, or substitute broccoli or cauliflower florets for the carrot or zucchini. Instead of parsley, sprinkle other fresh herbs over the vegetables.

CHOICES/EXCHANGES: 1 Nonstarchy Vegetable | 1 Fat
BASIC NUTRITIONAL VALUES: Calories 80 | Calories from Fat 30 | **Total Fat** 3.5 g | Saturated Fat 0.5 g | Trans Fat 0.0 g | **Cholesterol** 0 mg | **Sodium** 130 mg | **Potassium** 320 mg | **Total Carbohydrate** 10 g | Dietary Fiber 3 g | Sugars 5 g | **Protein** 2 g | **Phosphorus** 50 mg

Vegetarian Main Dishes and Whole Grains

Fried Sweet Potato Salad with Goat Cheese

SERVES: 4 | SERVING SIZE: 2 CUPS
PREP TIME: 15 MINUTES PLUS 10 MINUTES COOLING TIME | COOK TIME: 25 MINUTES

1 medium sweet potato, peeled and cut into 1-inch cubes

Nonstick cooking spray

6 cups spring mix lettuce

3 cups fresh spinach leaves, stems removed

¼ cup chopped pecans, toasted

1 medium apple, unpeeled, cored and thinly sliced

1 hard-cooked egg, chopped

2 tablespoons flaxseed

1 tablespoon Dijon mustard

2 tablespoons balsamic vinegar

1 tablespoon olive oil

2 tablespoons goat cheese crumbles

1 Place the sweet potato cubes in the air fryer basket. Spray the sweet potato cubes with nonstick cooking spray for 6 seconds.

2 Set the temperature to 400°F and air fry for about 25 minutes or until the potatoes are tender and crisp around the edges, shaking the air fryer basket every 10 minutes. Allow to cool for about 10 minutes before adding to salad.

3 While potatoes are air frying, make the salad. Place the spring lettuce and spinach into a large salad bowl. Add pecans, apple slices, egg, and sweet potato. Sprinkle with the flaxseed.

4 In a small bowl, whisk together the mustard and balsamic vinegar. Add the olive oil and whisk until blended well. Pour the dressing over the greens and toss gently. Sprinkle with the goat cheese crumbles. Serve immediately.

CHOICES/EXCHANGES: ½ Starch | ½ Carbohydrate | 1 Medium-Fat Protein | 1 ½ Fat
BASIC NUTRITIONAL VALUES: Calories 220 | Calories from Fat 130 | **Total Fat** 14.0 g | Saturated Fat 2.2 g | Trans Fat 0.0 g | **Cholesterol** 50 mg | **Sodium** 180 mg | **Potassium** 520 mg | **Total Carbohydrate** 19 g | Dietary Fiber 5 g | Sugars 8 g | **Protein** 6 g | **Phosphorus** 135 mg

Vegetable Calzones

SERVES: 4 | SERVING SIZE: 1 CALZONE | PREP TIME: 13 MINUTES | COOK TIME: 15–17 MINUTES

1 tablespoon olive oil
½ cup chopped onion
1 clove garlic
1 cup chopped broccoli
½ cup chopped cauliflower
1 cup fresh spinach leaves, stems removed
1 teaspoon salt-free Italian seasoning

1 cup part-skim shredded mozzarella cheese
2 tablespoons shredded Parmesan cheese
¼ cup flaxseed
6 ounces store-bought whole-wheat pizza dough

1 Preheat the air fryer, with the air fryer basket in place, to 400°F.

2 Heat the olive oil in a medium skillet over medium–high heat. Add the onion and cook for about 3 minutes. Stir in the garlic, broccoli, and cauliflower and cook for about 3 minutes. Add the spinach and Italian seasoning and cook an additional minute. Remove from the heat.

3 Add the mozzarella, Parmesan, and flaxseed to the vegetables.

4 On a lightly floured surface, roll the dough until very thin and about 12½ × 12½ inches. Cut the dough in half lengthwise and crosswise to get 4 equal pieces. Place about ½ cup filling on each dough piece. Gather the dough to cover filling and crimp to seal.

5 Place calzones in the air fryer basket. Air fry for 8–10 minutes until the dough is golden brown and cooked through. Serve warm.

CHOICES/EXCHANGES: 1½ Starch | 1 Nonstarchy Vegetable | 1 Medium-Fat Protein | 1½ Fat
BASIC NUTRITIONAL VALUES: Calories 270 | Calories from Fat 130 | **Total Fat** 14.0 g | Saturated Fat 4.1 g | Trans Fat 0.0 g | **Cholesterol** 20 mg | **Sodium** 390 mg | **Potassium** 370 mg | **Total Carbohydrate** 26 g | Dietary Fiber 6 g | Sugars 2 g | **Protein** 14 g | **Phosphorus** 310 mg

Artichoke Bites with Marinara

SERVES: 4 | SERVING SIZE: ½ CUP ARTICHOKE BITES WITH 2 TABLESPOONS MARINARA SAUCE
PREP TIME: 12 MINUTES | COOK TIME: 9–11 MINUTES

2   large egg whites, beaten
1½ cups whole-wheat panko
    bread crumbs
2   tablespoons flaxseed

2   cups frozen artichoke hearts,
    quartered, thawed
Nonstick cooking spray
½   cup marinara or meatless
    spaghetti sauce

1 Preheat the air fryer, with the air fryer basket in place, to 400°F.

2 Place the egg whites in a medium bowl. Combine the panko and flaxseed in a shallow dish.

3 Pat the artichoke hearts dry with paper towels. Dip the artichoke hearts in the egg-white mixture, allowing any excess to drain back into the bowl, then place in the panko mixture to coat. Set on a wire rack. Repeat with all artichoke pieces.

4 Arrange the coated artichokes in a single layer in the air fryer basket. Spray with nonstick cooking spray for 2 seconds. Air fry for 9–11 minutes until crispy and browning around the edges. Serve warm with the marinara sauce as a dip.

> **TIP**
> Do not crowd the artichokes. Many air fryer baskets can comfortably hold the artichokes, but others cannot. If your air fryer basket is smaller, it is better to cook half of the artichokes, then repeat with the remaining artichokes.

CHOICES/EXCHANGES: 1 ½ Starch | 2 Nonstarchy Vegetable | ½ Fat
BASIC NUTRITIONAL VALUES: Calories 190 | Calories from Fat 35 | **Total Fat** 4.0 g | Saturated Fat 0.5 g | Trans Fat 0.0 g | **Cholesterol** 0 mg | **Sodium** 250 mg | **Potassium** 430 mg | **Total Carbohydrate** 30 g | Dietary Fiber 10 g | Sugars 4 g | **Protein** 9 g | **Phosphorus** 135 mg

Mediterranean Stuffed Eggplant

SERVES: 2 | **SERVING SIZE:** ½ EGGPLANT | **PREP TIME:** 12 MINUTES | **COOK TIME:** 31–34 MINUTES

1 tablespoon olive oil
¼ cup chopped onions
2 cloves garlic, minced
¼ cup quick-cooking barley, uncooked
1 tablespoon dried oregano leaves
¼ teaspoon salt

¼ teaspoon coarse ground black pepper
½ cup water
1 medium (1-pound) eggplant
Nonstick cooking spray
¼ cup reduced-fat feta cheese crumbles

1 Heat the oil in a medium saucepan over medium-high heat. Stir in the onions and cook, stirring frequently, for 3 minutes. Stir in the garlic and cook for 30 seconds. Stir in the barley and cook for 2 minutes or until the barley is lightly toasted, stirring frequently. Stir in the oregano, salt, and pepper. Stir in the water. Cover, reduce the heat to a simmer, and cook for 10 minutes or until the barley is just tender and the water has been absorbed, stirring frequently. Remove from the heat and set aside.

2 Cut the eggplant in half lengthwise. Using the tip of a sharp knife, cut out the center portion of the eggplant, leaving a shell about ½ inch thick. Chop the removed eggplant into ½-inch pieces. Stir the chopped eggplant into the barley mixture.

3 If necessary, very thinly slice off an edge of the eggplant so each half rests flat with the cut side up. (Use caution not to cut through the eggplant shell.) Spray the cut sides of the eggplant with nonstick cooking spray for 1 second.

4 Spoon the barley mixture into the eggplant shells, mounding slightly. Spray the top of each with nonstick cooking spray for an additional 1 second. Place both eggplant halves into the air fryer basket. Set the temperature to 380°F and air fry for 14–16 minutes or until golden and eggplant is tender. Top each eggplant half with feta cheese. Air fry for 2–3 minutes.

CHOICES/EXCHANGES: 1 Starch | 4 Nonstarchy Vegetable | 2 Fat
BASIC NUTRITIONAL VALUES: Calories 260 | Calories from Fat 100 | **Total Fat** 11.0 g | Saturated Fat 2.5 g | Trans Fat 0.0 g | **Cholesterol** 5 mg | **Sodium** 470 mg | **Potassium** 380 mg | **Total Carbohydrate** 39 g | Dietary Fiber 9 g | Sugars 8 g | **Protein** 7 g | **Phosphorus** 130 mg

Crispy Quinoa Bites

SERVES: 4 | SERVING SIZE: 6 BITES
PREP TIME: 10 MINUTES PLUS 10 MINUTES COOLING TIME | COOK TIME: 51 MINUTES

1¼ cups quinoa, uncooked, drained and rinsed
2 large eggs
2 green onions, white and green portion, finely chopped
⅔ cup finely shredded carrot
2 cloves garlic, minced
¼ cup finely shredded Parmesan cheese
2 tablespoons minced fresh cilantro
2 tablespoons almond flour
½ teaspoon salt-free seasoning blend
¼ teaspoon coarse ground black pepper
1 teaspoon olive oil
Nonstick cooking spray

1 Cook the quinoa according to package directions, without added salt or fat, until done. Set aside to cool for about 10 minutes.

2 In a large bowl, whisk the eggs lightly. Stir in the green onions, carrot, garlic, Parmesan cheese, cilantro, almond flour, seasoning blend, pepper, and olive oil. Stir in the cooled quinoa.

> **TIP**
> For many air fryers, these are best cooked in 3 batches so as not to crowd the bites.

3 Spray the air fryer basket with nonstick cooking spray. Using wet hands, scoop about 2 tablespoons quinoa mixture and shape into a ball. Place about one third of the quinoa bites in the air fryer basket in a single layer so they are not touching. Spray for 1 second with nonstick cooking spray.

4 Set the air fryer at 375°F and air fry for 12 minutes or until quinoa bites are golden and crispy. Remove the bites from the air fryer basket. Repeat with the remaining quinoa mixture, cooking in two batches.

CHOICES/EXCHANGES: 2 ½ Starch | 1 Lean Protein | 1 Fat
BASIC NUTRITIONAL VALUES: Calories 280 | Calories from Fat 80 | **Total Fat** 9.0 g | Saturated Fat 1.9 g | Trans Fat 0.0 g | **Cholesterol** 50 mg | **Sodium** 100 mg | **Potassium** 430 mg | **Total Carbohydrate** 40 g | Dietary Fiber 5 g | Sugars 5 g | **Protein** 12 g | **Phosphorus** 325 mg

Stuffed Green Peppers

SERVES: 4 | SERVING SIZE: 1 STUFFED PEPPER | PREP TIME: 12 MINUTES | COOK TIME: 25 MINUTES

4 small (4-ounce) green bell peppers
1 cup canned no-salt-added black beans, drained and rinsed
1 cup petite diced no-salt-added tomatoes, drained
¾ cup cooked brown rice
2 teaspoons chili powder

⅛ teaspoon salt
1 cup reduced-fat shredded Mexican-blend cheese, divided
2 tablespoons minced fresh cilantro, divided
Nonstick cooking spray
1½ teaspoons coarse ground cornmeal

1 Cut off the stem end and remove the seeds from the green peppers.

2 In a medium bowl, stir together the black beans, tomatoes, brown rice, chili powder, salt, ¾ cup cheese, and 1 tablespoon cilantro. Spoon the mixture into the peppers. Set the peppers upright in the air fryer basket. Spray the peppers with nonstick cooking spray for 1 second. Set the temperature to 350°F and air fry for 20 minutes.

3 Spoon the remaining cheese on top of each pepper, then sprinkle lightly with the cornmeal. Air fry an additional 5 minutes or until the cheese is melted and the peppers are tender.

4 Sprinkle with remaining cilantro just before serving.

CHOICES/EXCHANGES: 1½ Starch | 1 Nonstarchy Vegetable | 1 Lean Protein | 1 Fat
BASIC NUTRITIONAL VALUES: Calories 220 | Calories from Fat 60 | **Total Fat** 7.0 g | Saturated Fat 3.8 g | Trans Fat 0.0 g | **Cholesterol** 15 mg | **Sodium** 310 mg | **Potassium** 550 mg | **Total Carbohydrate** 29 g | Dietary Fiber 6 g | Sugars 5 g | **Protein** 14 g | **Phosphorus** 280 mg

Crispy Cauliflower Street Tacos

SERVES: 4 | SERVING SIZE: 2 TACOS (EACH TACO MADE WITH 1 TORTILLA, ⅓ CUP CAULIFLOWER, 2 TABLESPOONS CHEESE, ABOUT 2 TEASPOONS YOGURT SAUCE, AND 1 TEASPOON SALSA)
PREP TIME: 15 MINUTES | COOK TIME: 10–16 MINUTES

4 cups bite-size cauliflower florets	Grated zest of ½ lime
1 tablespoon olive oil	1 teaspoon fresh lime juice
2 teaspoons chili powder	8 low-fat corn tortillas, each about 6 inches in diameter, warmed
1 teaspoon cumin	
½ teaspoon garlic powder	1 cup reduced-fat shredded cheddar cheese
⅛ teaspoon salt	
⅓ cup plain fat-free Greek yogurt	2 radishes, thinly sliced
2 tablespoons minced fresh cilantro	1 avocado, pitted, peeled, and sliced
	8 teaspoons salsa

1 Place the cauliflower in a bowl and drizzle with the olive oil. Season with the chili powder, cumin, garlic powder, and salt, and toss to season evenly.

2 Place about half of the cauliflower in the air fryer basket. Set the temperature to 400°F and air fry for 3–4 minutes. Shake the air fryer basket. Air fry for an additional 2–4 minutes or until the cauliflower is tender. Remove the cooked cauliflower and set aside; keep warm. Repeat with the remaining cauliflower.

3 While the cauliflower is air frying, mix together the yogurt, cilantro, lime zest, and lime juice in a small bowl. Set aside.

4 To assemble, spoon about ½ cup cauliflower down the center of each tortilla. Top each with about 1 tablespoon yogurt sauce and 2 tablespoons cheese. Garnish with radish slices and avocado slices. Drizzle with 1 teaspoon salsa, then fold the tortilla over loosely to make a taco.

CHOICES/EXCHANGES: 1 ½ Starch | 2 Nonstarchy Vegetable | 1 Medium-Fat Protein | 2 Fat
BASIC NUTRITIONAL VALUES: Calories 340 | Calories from Fat 150 | **Total Fat** 17.0 g | Saturated Fat 5.2 g | Trans Fat 0.0 g | **Cholesterol** 15 mg | **Sodium** 430 mg | **Potassium** 790 mg | **Total Carbohydrate** 37 g | Dietary Fiber 9 g | Sugars 5 g | **Protein** 16 g | **Phosphorus** 445 mg

Eggplant Parmesan with Basil-Tomato Topping

SERVES: 2 | SERVING SIZE: 1/2 EGGPLANT OR ABOUT 1 1/4 CUPS EGGPLANT SLICES
PREP TIME: 10 MINUTES | COOK TIME: 17–18 MINUTES

1 medium (1-pound) eggplant, about 8 inches long, not peeled	Nonstick cooking spray
2 large egg whites, beaten	1/4 cup marinara sauce
1 cup whole-wheat panko bread crumbs	1/4 cup fat-free shredded mozzarella cheese
	1/4 cup fresh basil leaves, cut into thin strips

1 Cut the eggplant into 3/4-inch slices. Dip the eggplant into egg whites, allowing excess to drip back into the bowl, and then into the panko bread crumbs, to coat. Place on a wire rack.

2 Preheat the air fryer, with the air fryer basket in place, to 400°F.

3 Spray the air fryer basket with nonstick cooking spray for 1 second. Spray the eggplant slices with nonstick cooking spray for 2 seconds. Arrange the eggplant in a single layer in the air fryer basket. Air fry for 8 minutes. Turn the eggplant. Air fry for an additional 8 minutes, or until the eggplant is tender.

4 Preheat the oven to broil. Place the cooked eggplant on a baking sheet. Divide the marinara between the eggplant slices. Divide the mozzarella between the eggplant slices. Broil about 1–2 minutes or until the cheese melts.

5 Transfer to serving platter and sprinkle with basil. Serve warm.

CHOICES/EXCHANGES: 1 1/2 Starch | 3 Nonstarchy Vegetable | 1 Lean Protein
BASIC NUTRITIONAL VALUES: Calories 220 | Calories from Fat 20 | **Total Fat** 2.5 g | Saturated Fat 0.3 g | Trans Fat 0.0 g | **Cholesterol** 0 mg | **Sodium** 350 mg | **Potassium** 480 mg | **Total Carbohydrate** 39 g | Dietary Fiber 8 g | Sugars 10 g | **Protein** 13 g | **Phosphorus** 155 mg

Balsamic–Glazed Vegetables on Couscous

SERVES: 4 | SERVING SIZE: 1 CUP VEGETABLES, ¼ CUP COOKED COUSCOUS, AND 1 TABLESPOON FETA CHEESE
PREP TIME: 10 MINUTES | COOK TIME: 30 MINUTES

2	medium carrots, sliced ½ inch thick	¼	teaspoon salt-free seasoning blend
1	medium (10-ounce) sweet potato, not peeled, sliced about ¼ inch thick	¼	teaspoon coarse ground black pepper
½	medium onion, sliced about ¼ inch thick	¼	cup pine nuts
		¾	cup whole-wheat couscous, not cooked
1	medium zucchini, not peeled, sliced in half lengthwise, then cut into 1-inch pieces	2	tablespoons balsamic vinegar
		¼	cup reduced-fat feta cheese
2	tablespoons olive oil, divided	1	tablespoon minced fresh flat-leaf (Italian) parsley

CHOICES/EXCHANGES: 2 ½ Starch | 1 Nonstarchy Vegetable | 2 ½ Fat
BASIC NUTRITIONAL VALUES: **Calories** 340 | Calories from Fat 130 | **Total Fat** 14.0 g | Saturated Fat 2.1 g | Trans Fat 0.0 g | **Cholesterol** 14 mg | **Sodium** 135 mg | **Potassium** 650 mg | **Total Carbohydrate** 46 g | Dietary Fiber 7 g | Sugars 9 g | **Protein** 10 g | **Phosphorus** 200 mg

1 Place the sliced carrots, sweet potato, onion, and zucchini in a mixing bowl. Drizzle with 1 tablespoon olive oil and sprinkle with seasoning blend and pepper; toss to coat the vegetables evenly. Spoon the vegetables into the air fryer basket.

2 Set the temperature to 375°F and air fry for 15 minutes. Stir the vegetables and air fry an additional 10 minutes or until the vegetables are almost tender. Sprinkle with the pine nuts and air fry for 5 minutes or until the vegetables are tender and the pine nuts are toasted.

3 While the vegetables are cooking, prepare the couscous according to the package directions, without added salt or fat. Stir and fluff the couscous, and place in a serving bowl. Top with the roasted vegetables and pine nuts.

4 Mix together the balsamic vinegar and the remaining 1 tablespoon olive oil. Drizzle the balsamic mixture over the vegetables and couscous, and toss to coat evenly. Sprinkle with the feta cheese and parsley.

Grilled Cheese Spinach Sandwich

SERVES: 1 | SERVING SIZE: 1 SANDWICH | PREP TIME: 5 MINUTES | COOK TIME: 8–10 MINUTES

2   slices reduced-calorie whole-wheat bread

1   teaspoon reduced-fat whipped tub margarine (such as I Can't Believe It's Not Butter Vegetable Oil Spread)

1   cup fresh spinach leaves, stems removed

2   very thin slices provolone or colby jack cheese (about ⅓ ounce per slice)

1 Spread one side of each slice of bread with margarine. Arrange spinach and cheese on one slice of bread, and top with a second slice of bread to form a sandwich, with buttered sides facing outside.

2 Place the sandwich in the air fryer basket. Set the temperature to 400°F and air fry for 8–10 minutes or until bread is toasted and cheese melts.

CHOICES/EXCHANGES: 1 ½ Starch | 1 Medium-Fat Protein
BASIC NUTRITIONAL VALUES: **Calories** 180 | Calories from Fat 70 | **Total Fat** 8.0 g | Saturated Fat 4.3 g | Trans Fat 0.0 g | **Cholesterol** 15 mg | **Sodium** 360 mg | **Potassium** 260 mg | **Total Carbohydrate** 19 g | Dietary Fiber 5 g | Sugars 2 g | **Protein** 11 g | **Phosphorus** 170 mg

Desserts

Apple Chips with Cinnamon Dip

SERVES: 2 | SERVING SIZE: ½ CUP APPLE CHIPS WITH 2 TABLESPOONS DIP
PREP TIME: 5 MINUTES | COOK TIME: 15 MINUTES

1 small (5-ounce), firm apple (such as a Granny Smith), not peeled, cored and quartered

1 tablespoon fresh lemon juice

1 teaspoon granulated sucralose sweetener (such as Splenda Blend for Baking)

1 teaspoon ground cinnamon, divided

2 tablespoons almond flour
Nonstick cooking spray

¼ cup plain fat-free Greek yogurt

1 tablespoon sugar-free maple-flavored breakfast syrup

1 Slice the apple quarters into very thin slices. Place the apple slices in a mixing bowl and drizzle with the lemon juice. Toss to coat the apple slices evenly, then drain.

2 In a small bowl, mix together the sweetener, ½ teaspoon cinnamon, and the almond flour. Toss the apple slices in the almond flour mixture, coating evenly. Place the apple slices in the air fryer basket, in a single layer if possible. If not, you may place a second layer on top. Spray with nonstick cooking spray for 1 second.

3 Set the temperature to 375°F and air fry for 15 minutes or until the apples are tender and the edges are crisp and golden, shaking the basket every 5 minutes.

4 While the apple is air frying, make the dip. In a small bowl, stir together the yogurt, syrup, and remaining ½ teaspoon cinnamon.

5 Serve the apple chips warm, with the cinnamon dip.

CHOICES/EXCHANGES: ½ Fruit | ½ Carbohydrate | 1 Fat
BASIC NUTRITIONAL VALUES: **Calories** 110 | Calories from Fat 40 | **Total Fat** 4.5 g | Saturated Fat 0.4 g | Trans Fat 0.0 g | Cholesterol 0 mg | **Sodium** 20 mg | **Potassium** 170 mg | **Total Carbohydrate** 15 g | Dietary Fiber 3 g | Sugars 11 g | **Protein** 5 g | **Phosphorus** 80 mg

Campfire Bananas

SERVES: 2 | SERVING SIZE: 1 FILLED BANANA | PREP TIME: 3 MINUTES | COOK TIME: 5–6 MINUTES

2   small (5½-ounce) bananas, each about 6–6⅞ inches long

1   tablespoon mini semisweet chocolate chips

1   tablespoon mini marshmallows

1   tablespoon bran cereal flakes

1 Slice the unpeeled bananas lengthwise along the middle, cutting through the fruit and making sure not to slice through the bottom peel. Open slightly to form a pocket. Divide the semisweet chips and the marshmallows between the two bananas, pushing them down into the banana. Sprinkle evenly with bran flakes.

> **TIPS**
> If the banana has a label on the peel, remove prior to frying.
>
> Bananas will blacken on the outside when cooked and will be soft in the inside.

2 Place the bananas in the air fryer basket, resting them on the side of the basket if need be to keep them upright. Set the temperature to 400°F and air fry for 5–6 minutes or until the bananas are soft to the touch and the chocolate and marshmallows have melted and toasted.

3 Let them cool for a few minutes, then serve. Use a spoon to scoop bites of the banana, with the filling, and enjoy.

CHOICES/EXCHANGES: 1½ Fruit | ½ Carbohydrate | ½ Fat
BASIC NUTRITIONAL VALUES: **Calories** 130 | Calories from Fat 20 | **Total Fat** 2.5 g | Saturated Fat 1.4 g | Trans Fat 0.0 g | Cholesterol 0 mg | **Sodium** 10 mg | **Potassium** 390 mg | **Total Carbohydrate** 30 g | Dietary Fiber 3 g | Sugars 17 g | **Protein** 2 g | **Phosphorus** 40 mg

Pecan Baked Apples

SERVES: 4 | SERVING SIZE: 1 APPLE | PREP TIME: 7 MINUTES | COOK TIME: 10–12 MINUTES

4 small (5-ounce) firm apples (such as Granny Smith), not peeled

1 tablespoon sugar-free maple-flavored breakfast syrup

2 tablespoons chopped pecans

2 tablespoons old-fashioned rolled oats

½ teaspoon ground cinnamon

1 tablespoon reduced-fat stick margarine (such as I Can't Believe It's Not Butter Stick Original, 79% Vegetable Oil Spread), melted

1 Cut off the stem and core the apples, not cutting through the bottom of the apple. Brush the inside of the apple cavity with the breakfast syrup.

2 Mix together the pecans, oats, cinnamon, and melted margarine. Spoon the pecan mixture into the cavity of each apple, mounding slightly. Place apples upright in the air fryer basket. Set the temperature to 350°F and air fry for 10–12 minutes or until tender.

> **TIP**
> For stuffed apples it is best to choose firm apples that hold their shape once baked. If you enjoy a tarter flavor, choose Granny Smith. For a sweeter flavor, choose Braeburn or Pink Lady.

CHOICES/EXCHANGES: 1 Fruit | ½ Carbohydrate | 1 Fat
BASIC NUTRITIONAL VALUES: Calories 130 | Calories from Fat 50 | **Total Fat** 6.0 g | Saturated Fat 1.2 g | Trans Fat 0.0 g | **Cholesterol** 0 mg | **Sodium** 30 mg | **Potassium** 170 mg | **Total Carbohydrate** 21 g | Dietary Fiber 4 g | Sugars 14 g | **Protein** 1 g | **Phosphorus** 35 mg

Tropical Pineapple

SERVES: 4 | SERVING SIZE: 3 PINEAPPLE STICKS | PREP TIME: 10 MINUTES | COOK TIME: 10–12 MINUTES

3 tablespoons unsweetened flaked coconut

6 tablespoons chopped almonds

½ fresh pineapple, peeled, cored, and cut into 12 (1-inch) sticks

1 Preheat the air fryer, with the air fryer basket in place, to 400°F.

2 Combine the coconut and almonds in shallow dish. Roll the pineapple sticks in the coconut mixture to lightly coat. Place the coated pineapple in the air fryer basket. Air fry for 10–12 minutes or until heated and coconut and nuts are toasted. Allow to cool slightly before serving. Serve warm.

CHOICES/EXCHANGES: 1 Fruit | 1½ Fat

BASIC NUTRITIONAL VALUES: Calories 130 | Calories from Fat 60 | **Total Fat** 7.0 g | Saturated Fat 2.5 g | Trans Fat 0.0 g | **Cholesterol** 0 mg | **Sodium** 0 mg | **Potassium** 180 mg | **Total Carbohydrate** 14 g | Dietary Fiber 3 g | Sugars 9 g | **Protein** 3 g | **Phosphorus** 60 mg

Peach Galette

SERVES: 4 | SERVING SIZE: ¼ GALETTE | PREP TIME: 15 MINUTES PLUS AT LEAST 10 MINUTES FOR DOUGH TO REST AND 10 MINUTES COOLING TIME | COOK TIME: 20–22 MINUTES

½ cup whole-wheat flour
¼ cup all-purpose flour
1½ teaspoons flaxseed meal
⅛ teaspoon salt
2½ tablespoons reduced-fat stick margarine (such as I Can't Believe It's Not Butter Stick Original, 79% Vegetable Oil Spread)
4–5 tablespoons cold water

2 medium (6-ounce) peaches, peeled, pitted, and sliced ½ inch thick
1 teaspoon granulated sucralose sweetener (such as Splenda Blend for Baking)
1 tablespoon apricot sugar-free all-fruit spread
1 tablespoon sliced almonds

1 In a mixing bowl, stir together the whole-wheat flour, all-purpose flour, flaxseed meal, and salt. Cut in the margarine with a pastry cutter or two knives until the mixture resembles coarse crumbs. Stir in 4 tablespoons water. (If needed to make the dough come together, add additional water.) Gather dough into a ball. Wrap in plastic wrap and refrigerate for at least 10 minutes or up to an hour.

2 Cut a 7-inch circle of parchment paper and place the circle on a lightly floured work surface. Lightly flour the top of the parchment paper.

3 Place the dough on the center of the parchment paper circle. Roll the dough over the parchment circle into an 8–9-inch circle, about ¼–½ inch thick.

CHOICES/EXCHANGES: 1 Starch | 1 Fruit | 1 ½ Fat
BASIC NUTRITIONAL VALUES: **Calories** 200 | Calories from Fat 80 | **Total Fat** 9.0 g | Saturated Fat 2.4 g | Trans Fat 0.0 g | **Cholesterol** 0 mg | **Sodium** 140 mg | **Potassium** 240 mg | **Total Carbohydrate** 28 g | Dietary Fiber 4 g | Sugars 9 g | **Protein** 4 g | **Phosphorus** 90 mg

4 Preheat the air fryer, with the air fryer basket in place, to 350°F.

5 Arrange the sliced peaches in the center of the pastry circle in a decorative pattern, leaving a 1-inch border all around the edges and layering as necessary. Sprinkle the peaches with the sweetener.

6 Put the all-fruit spread in a small, microwave-safe glass bowl. Microwave on high (100% power) for 15 seconds or until melted. Brush the peaches with the all-fruit spread. Sprinkle the almonds over the top. Gently fold the pastry edges up over the edges of the fruit. (Pastry will not cover the center.)

7 Leaving the galette on the parchment paper, and using a wide spatula, gently lift the galette into the basket. Note: If basket is deep, follow the tip to make two foil slings. Be careful as the air fryer basket will be hot. Air fry for 20–22 minutes or until crust is golden brown and peaches are tender.

8 Open the air fryer and allow the dessert to cool about 5 minutes before carefully removing the dessert from the air fryer basket. Using a wide, flexible spatula, slide it under the parchment paper and lift, or use the slings if available. Transfer to a wire rack. Allow to stand 5 more minutes. Slice, and serve warm.

TIP
To make foil slings, take a sheet of aluminum foil about 14–15 inches long. Fold it to make a strip about 2 inches wide. Repeat with a second sheet of foil. Place the strips criss-cross fashion across the bottom of the basket and leave foil extending up the sides. Place the parchment paper circle with the galette on top of the foil slings. The foil sling will still allow the air to circulate around the galette, but will help to safely lift it up out of the hot basket.

Roasted Nectarines

SERVES: 2 | SERVING SIZE: 1 NECTARINE | PREP TIME: 5 MINUTES | COOK TIME: 6–7 MINUTES

2 medium (6-ounce) nectarines, not peeled

Nonstick cooking spray

2 tablespoons chopped pecans

2 tablespoons old-fashioned rolled oats

1 tablespoon flaxseed

1 teaspoon granulated sucralose sweetener (such as Splenda Blend for Baking)

½ teaspoon ground cinnamon

1 Cut the nectarines in half and carefully remove the pit. Spray the cut side of each nectarine half with nonstick cooking spray for 1 second. Place the nectarines, cut side up, in the air fryer basket. Set the temperature to 350°F and air fry for 5 minutes.

2 While the nectarines are air frying, stir together the pecans, oats, flaxseed, sweetener, and cinnamon in a small bowl. Spoon the nut mixture over the cut side of each nectarine, mounding slightly. Spray each nectarine with nonstick cooking spray for 1 second. Air fry for an additional 1–2 minutes or until the nut mixture turns golden brown.

CHOICES/EXCHANGES: 1 Fruit | ½ Carbohydrate | 2 ½ Fat

BASIC NUTRITIONAL VALUES: Calories 210 | Calories from Fat 110 | **Total Fat** 12.0 g | Saturated Fat 1.0 g | Trans Fat 0.0 g | **Cholesterol** 0 mg | **Sodium** 5 mg | **Potassium** 400 mg | **Total Carbohydrate** 26 g | Dietary Fiber 6 g | Sugars 15 g | **Protein** 4 g | **Phosphorus** 115 mg

Roasted Pears with Almonds and Cream

SERVES: 4 | SERVING SIZE: 6 TABLESPOONS | PREP TIME: 5 MINUTES PLUS 5 MINUTES COOLING TIME | COOK TIME: 14 MINUTES

2	medium Bosc pears, peeled, quartered, and pitted
1	tablespoon fresh lemon juice
1	teaspoon granulated sucralose sweetener (such as Splenda Blend for Baking)
¼	cup slivered almonds, finely chopped
2	tablespoons whole-wheat panko bread crumbs
¼	teaspoon ground nutmeg
	Butter-flavored nonstick cooking spray
1	tablespoon fat-free sour cream
½	teaspoon vanilla extract

1 Cut each pear quarter into thirds. Place the pear slices in a 6-inch round baking pan (see Tip). Drizzle the pears with the lemon juice and toss gently to coat evenly. Sprinkle with the sweetener.

2 Place the filled, uncovered pan into the air fryer basket. Set the temperature to 375°F and air fry for 5 minutes.

3 While the pears are air frying, stir together the chopped almonds, panko bread crumbs, and nutmeg in a small bowl. Once pears are done frying, sprinkle the almond mixture over the pears. Spray with butter-flavored nonstick cooking spray for 2 seconds. Air fry for an additional 9 minutes or until the crumbs are toasted and golden. Open the air fryer and let dessert cool about 5 minutes before carefully removing the pan from the air fryer basket.

4 Stir together the sour cream and vanilla. Drizzle the sour cream mixture over the pears. Serve warm.

CHOICES/EXCHANGES: 1 Fruit | 1 Fat

BASIC NUTRITIONAL VALUES: Calories 110 | Calories from Fat 40 | **Total Fat** 4.5 g | Saturated Fat 0.4 g | Trans Fat 0.0 g | **Cholesterol** 0 mg | **Sodium** 10 mg | **Potassium** 150 mg | **Total Carbohydrate** 16 g | Dietary Fiber 3 g | Sugars 9 g | **Protein** 2 g | **Phosphorus** 50 mg

TIPS

A small metal baking pan, about 6 inches in diameter and about 1¾ inches deep, works well in most air fryers. As an alternative, you could use a 6-inch (individual size) metal pie pan or 3-cup oven-safe metal mixing bowl. Double-check the fit before you begin the recipe. Fill the pan no more than about ¾ full. Do not cover the pan while air frying. Once the air frying is done, carefully remove the pan with hot pan holders. Use caution as the pan and the air fryer basket will be very hot.

A foil sling will assist when removing a hot pan. To make foil slings, take a sheet of aluminum foil about 14–15 inches long. Fold it to make a strip about 2 inches wide. Repeat with a second sheet of foil. Place the strips criss-cross fashion across the bottom of the basket and leave foil extending up the sides. Place the filled pan on top of the foil slings. The foil sling will still allow the air to circulate around the pan, but will help to safely lift it up out of the hot basket.

Berry Crumble

SERVES: 4 | SERVING SIZE: ABOUT 7 TABLESPOONS
PREP TIME: 5 MINUTES PLUS 5 MINUTES COOLING TIME
COOK TIME: 18 MINUTES

1   cup blueberries
½   cup blackberries
½   cup raspberries
1   tablespoon fresh lemon juice
1   tablespoon strawberry all-fruit spread
2   tablespoons granulated sucralose sweetener
      (such as Splenda Blend for Baking)
½   teaspoon ground cinnamon
½   cup reduced-fat granola (such as Special K
      Touch of Honey granola)
Butter-flavored nonstick cooking spray

1 Place the berries in a 6-inch round baking pan
(see Tip).

2 In a small bowl, stir together the lemon juice,
all-fruit spread, sweetener, and cinnamon. Spoon
the lemon juice mixture over the fruit and very
gently stir to coat the berries evenly.

3 Place the filled, uncovered pan into the air fryer
basket. Set the temperature to 350°F and air fry for
10 minutes.

4 Sprinkle the granola over the berries. Spray the
granola with the butter-flavored nonstick cooking
spray for 2 seconds. Air fry for an additional 8 minutes or until the berries are bubbling and the granola
is toasted. Open the air fryer and allow the dessert
to cool about 5 minutes before carefully removing
the pan from the air fryer basket. Serve warm.

CHOICES/EXCHANGES: ½ Starch | 1 Fruit | ½ Carbohydrate
BASIC NUTRITIONAL VALUES: Calories 130 | Calories from Fat 15 | **Total Fat** 1.5 g | Saturated
Fat 0.2 g | Trans Fat 0.0 g | **Cholesterol** 0 mg | **Sodium** 35 mg |
Potassium 125 mg | **Total Carbohydrate** 28 g | Dietary Fiber
4 g | Sugars 16 g | **Protein** 2 g | **Phosphorus** 45 mg

TIPS

Select your favorite
berries for this dessert.
You might make it with all
blueberries, or with your
favorite combination.

A small metal baking pan,
about 6 inches in diameter,
and about 1 ¾ inches deep,
works well in most air
fryers. As an alternative,
you could use a 6-inch
(individual size) metal pie
pan or 3-cup oven-safe
metal mixing bowl.
Double-check the fit before
you begin the recipe. Fill
the pan no more than
about ¾ full. Do not cover
the pan while air frying.
Once the air frying is done,
carefully remove the pan
with hot pan holders. Use
caution as the pan and
the air fryer basket will be
very hot.

A foil sling will assist
when removing a hot
pan. To make foil slings,
take a sheet of aluminum
foil about 14–15 inches
long. Fold it to make a
strip about 2 inches wide.
Repeat with a second sheet
of foil. Place the strips,
criss-cross fashion across
the bottom of the basket
and leave foil extending
up the sides. Place the
filled pan on top of the foil
slings. The foil sling will still
allow the air to circulate
around the pan, but will
help to safely lift it up out
of the hot basket.

Index